Mometrix
TEST PREPARATION

Secrets of the

ARDMS®

Vascular Technology Exam Study Guide

ARDMS and American Registry for Diagnostic Medical Sonography are registered trademarks of Intelios, Inc. The American Registry for Diagnostic Medical Sonography, Inc. (ARDMS) does not endorse this product nor is the ARDMS affiliated in any way with the owner or any content related to this product.

AF901632

DEAR FUTURE EXAM SUCCESS STORY

First of all, **THANK YOU** for purchasing Mometrix study materials!

Second, congratulations! You are one of the few determined test-takers who are committed to doing whatever it takes to excel on your exam. **You have come to the right place.** We developed these study materials with one goal in mind: to deliver you the information you need in a format that's concise and easy to use.

In addition to optimizing your guide for the content of the test, we've outlined our recommended steps for breaking down the preparation process into small, attainable goals so you can make sure you stay on track.

We've also analyzed the entire test-taking process, identifying the most common pitfalls and showing how you can overcome them and be ready for any curveball the test throws you.

Standardized testing is one of the biggest obstacles on your road to success, which only increases the importance of doing well in the high-pressure, high-stakes environment of test day. Your results on this test could have a significant impact on your future, and this guide provides the information and practical advice to help you achieve your full potential on test day.

Your success is our success

We would love to hear from you! If you would like to share the story of your exam success or if you have any questions or comments in regard to our products, please contact us at **800-673-8175** or **support@mometrix.com**.

Thanks again for your business and we wish you continued success!

Sincerely,
The Mometrix Test Preparation Team

Need more help? Check out our flashcards at:
http://mometrixflashcards.com/ARDMS

Copyright © 2026 by Mometrix Media LLC. All rights reserved.
Written and edited by the Mometrix Exam Secrets Test Prep Team
Printed in the United States of America

TABLE OF CONTENTS

Introduction

Thank you for purchasing this resource! You have made the choice to prepare yourself for a test that could have a huge impact on your future, and this guide is designed to help you be fully ready for test day. Obviously, it's important to have a solid understanding of the test material, but you also need to be prepared for the unique environment and stressors of the test, so that you can perform to the best of your abilities.

For this purpose, the first section that appears in this guide is the **Secret Keys**. We've devoted countless hours to meticulously researching what works and what doesn't, and we've boiled down our findings to the five most impactful steps you can take to improve your performance on the test. We start at the beginning with study planning and move through the preparation process, all the way to the testing strategies that will help you get the most out of what you know when you're finally sitting in front of the test.

We recommend that you start preparing for your test as far in advance as possible. However, if you've bought this guide as a last-minute study resource and only have a few days before your test, we recommend that you skip over the first two Secret Keys since they address a long-term study plan.

If you struggle with **test anxiety**, we strongly encourage you to check out our recommendations for how you can overcome it. Test anxiety is a formidable foe, but it can be beaten, and we want to make sure you have the tools you need to defeat it.

Copyright © Mometrix Media. You have been licensed one copy of this document for personal use only. Any other reproduction or redistribution is strictly prohibited. All rights reserved.
This content is provided for test preparation purposes only and does not imply an endorsement by Mometrix of any particular political, scientific, or religious point of view.

Secret Key 1: Plan Big, Study Small

There's a lot riding on your performance. If you want to ace this test, you're going to need to keep your skills sharp and the material fresh in your mind. You need a plan that lets you review everything you need to know while still fitting in your schedule. We'll break this strategy down into three categories.

Information Organization

Start with the information you already have: the official test outline. From this, you can make a complete list of all the concepts you need to cover before the test. Organize these concepts into groups that can be studied together, and create a list of any related vocabulary you need to learn so you can brush up on any difficult terms. You'll want to keep this vocabulary list handy once you actually start studying since you may need to add to it along the way.

Time Management

Once you have your set of study concepts, decide how to spread them out over the time you have left before the test. Break your study plan into small, clear goals so you have a manageable task for each day and know exactly what you're doing. Then just focus on one small step at a time. When you manage your time this way, you don't need to spend hours at a time studying. Studying a small block of content for a short period each day helps you retain information better and avoid stressing over how much you have left to do. You can relax knowing that you have a plan to cover everything in time. In order for this strategy to be effective though, you have to start studying early and stick to your schedule. Avoid the exhaustion and futility that comes from last-minute cramming!

Study Environment

The environment you study in has a big impact on your learning. Studying in a coffee shop, while probably more enjoyable, is not likely to be as fruitful as studying in a quiet room. It's important to keep distractions to a minimum. You're only planning to study for a short block of time, so make the most of it. Don't pause to check your phone or get up to find a snack. It's also important to **avoid multitasking**. Research has consistently shown that multitasking will make your studying dramatically less effective. Your study area should also be comfortable and well-lit so you don't have the distraction of straining your eyes or sitting on an uncomfortable chair.

Copyright © Mometrix Media. You have been licensed one copy of this document for personal use only. Any other reproduction or redistribution is strictly prohibited. All rights reserved.
This content is provided for test preparation purposes only and does not imply an endorsement by Mometrix of any particular political, scientific, or religious point of view.

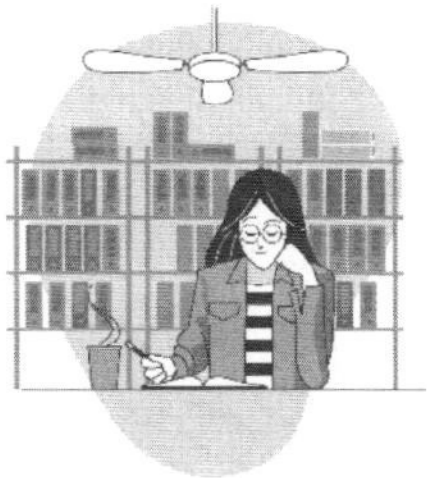

The time of day you study is also important. You want to be rested and alert. Don't wait until just before bedtime. Study when you'll be most likely to comprehend and remember. Even better, if you know what time of day your test will be, set that time aside for study. That way your brain will be used to working on that subject at that specific time and you'll have a better chance of recalling information.

Finally, it can be helpful to team up with others who are studying for the same test. Your actual studying should be done in as isolated an environment as possible, but the work of organizing the information and setting up the study plan can be divided up. In between study sessions, you can discuss with your teammates the concepts that you're all studying and quiz each other on the details. Just be sure that your teammates are as serious about the test as you are. If you find that your study time is being replaced with social time, you might need to find a new team.

Copyright © Mometrix Media. You have been licensed one copy of this document for personal use only. Any other reproduction or redistribution is strictly prohibited. All rights reserved.
This content is provided for test preparation purposes only and does not imply an endorsement by Mometrix of any particular political, scientific, or religious point of view.

Secret Key 2: Make Your Studying Count

You're devoting a lot of time and effort to preparing for this test, so you want to be absolutely certain it will pay off. This means doing more than just reading the content and hoping you can remember it on test day. It's important to make every minute of study count. There are two main areas you can focus on to make your studying count.

Retention

It doesn't matter how much time you study if you can't remember the material. You need to make sure you are retaining the concepts. To check your retention of the information you're learning, try recalling it at later times with minimal prompting. Try carrying around flashcards and glance at one or two from time to time or ask a friend who's also studying for the test to quiz you.

To enhance your retention, look for ways to put the information into practice so that you can apply it rather than simply recalling it. If you're using the information in practical ways, it will be much easier to remember. Similarly, it helps to solidify a concept in your mind if you're not only reading it to yourself but also explaining it to someone else. Ask a friend to let you teach them about a concept you're a little shaky on (or speak aloud to an imaginary audience if necessary). As you try to summarize, define, give examples, and answer your friend's questions, you'll understand the concepts better and they will stay with you longer. Finally, step back for a big picture view and ask yourself how each piece of information fits with the whole subject. When you link the different concepts together and see them working together as a whole, it's easier to remember the individual components.

Finally, practice showing your work on any multi-step problems, even if you're just studying. Writing out each step you take to solve a problem will help solidify the process in your mind, and you'll be more likely to remember it during the test.

Modality

Modality simply refers to the means or method by which you study. Choosing a study modality that fits your own individual learning style is crucial. No two people learn best in exactly the same way, so it's important to know your strengths and use them to your advantage.

Copyright © Mometrix Media. You have been licensed one copy of this document for personal use only. Any other reproduction or redistribution is strictly prohibited. All rights reserved.
This content is provided for test preparation purposes only and does not imply an endorsement by Mometrix of any particular political, scientific, or religious point of view.

For example, if you learn best by visualization, focus on visualizing a concept in your mind and draw an image or a diagram. Try color-coding your notes, illustrating them, or creating symbols that will trigger your mind to recall a learned concept. If you learn best by hearing or discussing information, find a study partner who learns the same way or read aloud to yourself. Think about how to put the information in your own words. Imagine that you are giving a lecture on the topic and record yourself so you can listen to it later.

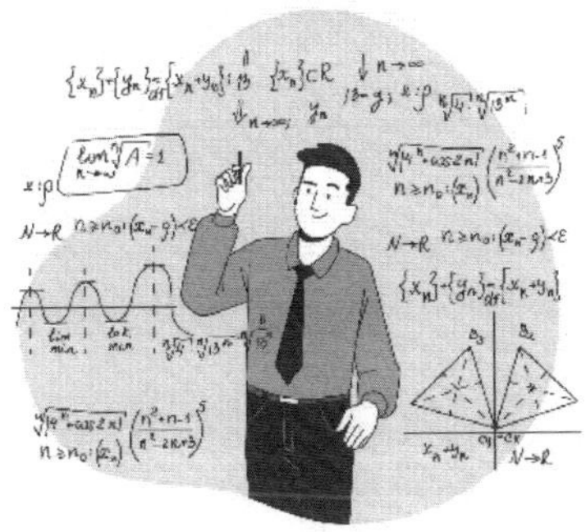

For any learning style, flashcards can be helpful. Organize the information so you can take advantage of spare moments to review. Underline key words or phrases. Use different colors for different categories. Mnemonic devices (such as creating a short list in which every item starts with the same letter) can also help with retention. Find what works best for you and use it to store the information in your mind most effectively and easily.

Copyright © Mometrix Media. You have been licensed one copy of this document for personal use only. Any other reproduction or redistribution is strictly prohibited. All rights reserved.
This content is provided for test preparation purposes only and does not imply an endorsement by Mometrix of any particular political, scientific, or religious point of view.

Secret Key 3: Practice the Right Way

Your success on test day depends not only on how many hours you put into preparing, but also on whether you prepared the right way. It's good to check along the way to see if your studying is paying off. One of the most effective ways to do this is by taking practice tests to evaluate your progress. Practice tests are useful because they show exactly where you need to improve. Every time you take a practice test, pay special attention to these three groups of questions:

- The questions you got wrong
- The questions you had to guess on, even if you guessed right
- The questions you found difficult or slow to work through

This will show you exactly what your weak areas are, and where you need to devote more study time. Ask yourself why each of these questions gave you trouble. Was it because you didn't understand the material? Was it because you didn't remember the vocabulary? Do you need more repetitions on this type of question to build speed and confidence? Dig into those questions and figure out how you can strengthen your weak areas as you go back to review the material.

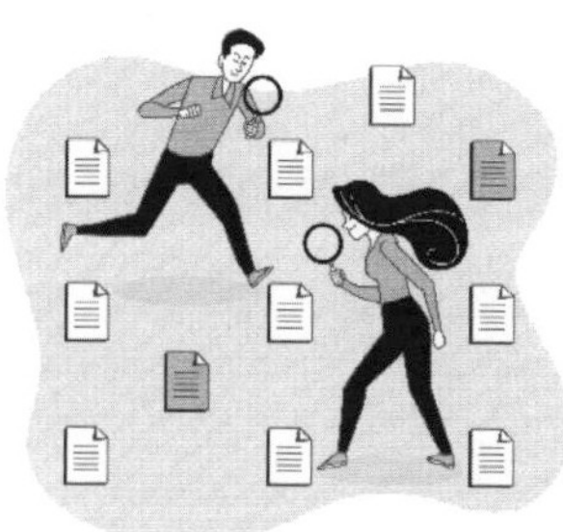

Additionally, many practice tests have a section explaining the answer choices. It can be tempting to read the explanation and think that you now have a good understanding of the concept. However, an explanation likely only covers part of the question's broader context. Even if the explanation makes perfect sense, **go back and investigate** every concept related to the question until you're positive you have a thorough understanding.

As you go along, keep in mind that the practice test is just that: practice. Memorizing these questions and answers will not be very helpful on the actual test because it is unlikely to have any of the same exact questions. If you only know the right answers to the sample questions, you won't be prepared for the real thing. **Study the concepts** until you understand them fully, and then you'll be able to answer any question that shows up on the test.

It's important to wait on the practice tests until you're ready. If you take a test on your first day of study, you may be overwhelmed by the amount of material covered and how much you need to learn. Work up to it gradually.

On test day, you'll need to be prepared for answering questions, managing your time, and using the test-taking strategies you've learned. It's a lot to balance, like a mental marathon that will have a big impact on your future. Like training for a marathon, you'll need to start slowly and work your way up. When test day arrives, you'll be ready.

Copyright © Mometrix Media. You have been licensed one copy of this document for personal use only. Any other reproduction or redistribution is strictly prohibited. All rights reserved.
This content is provided for test preparation purposes only and does not imply an endorsement by Mometrix of any particular political, scientific, or religious point of view.

Start with the strategies you've read in the first two Secret Keys—plan your course and study in the way that works best for you. If you have time, consider using multiple study resources to get different approaches to the same concepts. It can be helpful to see difficult concepts from more than one angle. Then find a good source for practice tests. Many times, the test website will suggest potential study resources or provide sample tests.

Practice Test Strategy

If you're able to find at least three practice tests, we recommend this strategy:

Untimed and Open-Book Practice

Take the first test with no time constraints and with your notes and study guide handy. Take your time and focus on applying the strategies you've learned.

Timed and Open-Book Practice

Take the second practice test open-book as well, but set a timer and practice pacing yourself to finish in time.

Timed and Closed-Book Practice

Take any other practice tests as if it were test day. Set a timer and put away your study materials. Sit at a table or desk in a quiet room, imagine yourself at the testing center, and answer questions as quickly and accurately as possible.

Keep repeating timed and closed-book tests on a regular basis until you run out of practice tests or it's time for the actual test. Your mind will be ready for the schedule and stress of test day, and you'll be able to focus on recalling the material you've learned.

Copyright © Mometrix Media. You have been licensed one copy of this document for personal use only. Any other reproduction or redistribution is strictly prohibited. All rights reserved.
This content is provided for test preparation purposes only and does not imply an endorsement by Mometrix of any particular political, scientific, or religious point of view.

Secret Key 4: Pace Yourself

Once you're fully prepared for the material on the test, your biggest challenge on test day will be managing your time. Just knowing that the clock is ticking can make you panic even if you have plenty of time left. Work on pacing yourself so you can build confidence against the time constraints of the exam. Pacing is a difficult skill to master, especially in a high-pressure environment, so **practice is vital**.

Set time expectations for your pace based on how much time is available. For example, if a section has 60 questions and the time limit is 30 minutes, you know you have to average 30 seconds or less per question in order to answer them all. Although 30 seconds is the hard limit, set 25 seconds per question as your goal, so you reserve extra time to spend on harder questions. When you budget extra time for the harder questions, you no longer have any reason to stress when those questions take longer to answer.

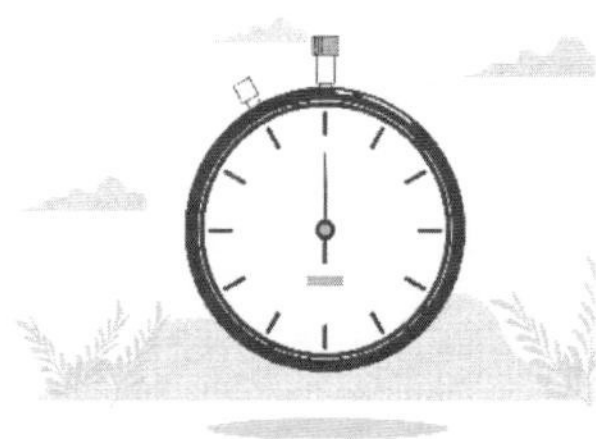

Don't let this time expectation distract you from working through the test at a calm, steady pace, but keep it in mind so you don't spend too much time on any one question. Recognize that taking extra time on one question you don't understand may keep you from answering two that you do understand later in the test. If your time limit for a question is up and you're still not sure of the answer, mark it and move on, and come back to it later if the time and the test format allow. If the testing format doesn't allow you to return to earlier questions, just make an educated guess; then put it out of your mind and move on.

On the easier questions, be careful not to rush. It may seem wise to hurry through them so you have more time for the challenging ones, but it's not worth missing one if you know the concept and just didn't take the time to read the question fully. Work efficiently but make sure you understand the question and have looked at all of the answer choices, since more than one may seem right at first.

Even if you're paying attention to the time, you may find yourself a little behind at some point. You should speed up to get back on track, but do so wisely. Don't panic; just take a few seconds less on each question until you're caught up. Don't guess without thinking, but do look through the answer choices and eliminate any you know are wrong. If you can get down to two choices, it is often worthwhile to guess from those. Once you've chosen an answer, move on and don't dwell on any that you skipped or had to hurry through. If a question was taking too long, chances are it was one of the harder ones, so you weren't as likely to get it right anyway.

Copyright © Mometrix Media. You have been licensed one copy of this document for personal use only. Any other reproduction or redistribution is strictly prohibited. All rights reserved.
This content is provided for test preparation purposes only and does not imply an endorsement by Mometrix of any particular political, scientific, or religious point of view.

On the other hand, if you find yourself getting ahead of schedule, it may be beneficial to slow down a little. The more quickly you work, the more likely you are to make a careless mistake that will affect your score. You've budgeted time for each question, so don't be afraid to spend that time. Practice an efficient but careful pace to get the most out of the time you have.

Copyright © Mometrix Media. You have been licensed one copy of this document for personal use only. Any other reproduction or redistribution is strictly prohibited. All rights reserved.
This content is provided for test preparation purposes only and does not imply an endorsement by Mometrix of any particular political, scientific, or religious point of view.

Secret Key 5: Have a Plan for Guessing

When you're taking the test, you may find yourself stuck on a question. Some of the answer choices seem better than others, but you don't see the one answer choice that is obviously correct. What do you do?

The scenario described above is very common, yet most test takers have not effectively prepared for it. Developing and practicing a plan for guessing may be one of the single most effective uses of your time as you get ready for the exam.

In developing your plan for guessing, there are three questions to address:

- When should you start the guessing process?
- How should you narrow down the choices?
- Which answer should you choose?

When to Start the Guessing Process

Unless your plan for guessing is to select C every time (which, despite its merits, is not what we recommend), you need to leave yourself enough time to apply your answer elimination strategies. Since you have a limited amount of time for each question, that means that if you're going to give yourself the best shot at guessing correctly, you have to decide quickly whether or not you will guess.

Of course, the best-case scenario is that you don't have to guess at all, so first, see if you can answer the question based on your knowledge of the subject and basic reasoning skills. Focus on the key words in the question and try to jog your memory of related topics. Give yourself a chance to bring the knowledge to mind, but once you realize that you don't have (or you can't access) the knowledge you need to answer the question, it's time to start the guessing process.

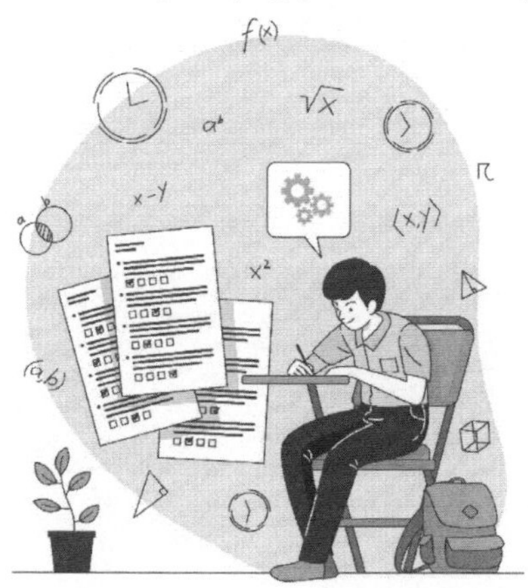

It's almost always better to start the guessing process too early than too late. It only takes a few seconds to remember something and answer the question from knowledge. Carefully eliminating wrong answer choices takes longer. Plus, going through the process of eliminating answer choices can actually help jog your memory.

Summary: Start the guessing process as soon as you decide that you can't answer the question based on your knowledge.

Copyright © Mometrix Media. You have been licensed one copy of this document for personal use only. Any other reproduction or redistribution is strictly prohibited. All rights reserved.
This content is provided for test preparation purposes only and does not imply an endorsement by Mometrix of any particular political, scientific, or religious point of view.

How to Narrow Down the Choices

The next chapter in this book (**Test-Taking Strategies**) includes a wide range of strategies for how to approach questions and how to look for answer choices to eliminate. You will definitely want to read those carefully, practice them, and figure out which ones work best for you. Here though, we're going to address a mindset rather than a particular strategy.

Your odds of guessing an answer correctly depend on how many options you are choosing from.

Number of options left	5	4	3	2	1
Odds of guessing correctly	20%	25%	33%	50%	100%

You can see from this chart just how valuable it is to be able to eliminate incorrect answers and make an educated guess, but there are two things that many test takers do that cause them to miss out on the benefits of guessing:

- Accidentally eliminating the correct answer
- Selecting an answer based on an impression

We'll look at the first one here, and the second one in the next section.

To avoid accidentally eliminating the correct answer, we recommend a thought exercise called **the $5 challenge**. In this challenge, you only eliminate an answer choice from contention if you are willing to bet $5 on it being wrong. Why $5? Five dollars is a small but not insignificant amount of money. It's an amount you could afford to lose but wouldn't want to throw away. And while losing $5 once might not hurt too much, doing it twenty times will set you back $100. In the same way, each small decision you make—eliminating a choice here, guessing on a question there—won't by itself impact your score very much, but when you put them all together, they can make a big difference. By holding each answer choice elimination decision to a higher standard, you can reduce the risk of accidentally eliminating the correct answer.

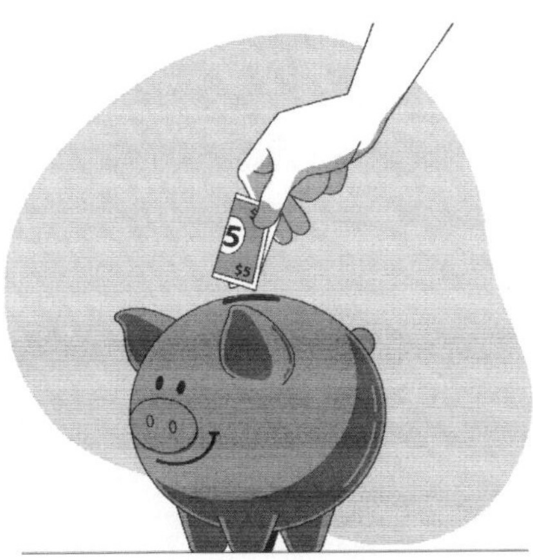

The $5 challenge can also be applied in a positive sense: If you are willing to bet $5 that an answer choice *is* correct, go ahead and mark it as correct.

Summary: Only eliminate an answer choice if you are willing to bet $5 that it is wrong.

Copyright © Mometrix Media. You have been licensed one copy of this document for personal use only. Any other reproduction or redistribution is strictly prohibited. All rights reserved.
This content is provided for test preparation purposes only and does not imply an endorsement by Mometrix of any particular political, scientific, or religious point of view.

Which Answer to Choose

You're taking the test. You've run into a hard question and decided you'll have to guess. You've eliminated all the answer choices you're willing to bet $5 on. Now you have to pick an answer. Why do we even need to talk about this? Why can't you just pick whichever one you feel like when the time comes?

The answer to these questions is that if you don't come into the test with a plan, you'll rely on your impression to select an answer choice, and if you do that, you risk falling into a trap. The test writers know that everyone who takes their test will be guessing on some of the questions, so they intentionally write wrong answer choices to seem plausible. You still have to pick an answer though, and if the wrong answer choices are designed to look right, how can you ever be sure that you're not falling for their trap? The best solution we've found to this dilemma is to take the decision out of your hands entirely. Here is the process we recommend:

Once you've eliminated any choices that you are confident (willing to bet $5) are wrong, select the first remaining choice as your answer.

Whether you choose to select the first remaining choice, the second, or the last, the important thing is that you use some preselected standard. Using this approach guarantees that you will not be enticed into selecting an answer choice that looks right, because you are not basing your decision on how the answer choices look.

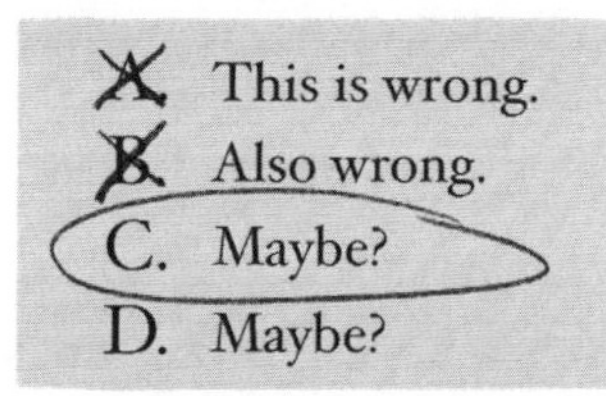

This is not meant to make you question your knowledge. Instead, it is to help you recognize the difference between your knowledge and your impressions. There's a huge difference between thinking an answer is right because of what you know, and thinking an answer is right because it looks or sounds like it should be right.

Summary: To ensure that your selection is appropriately random, make a predetermined selection from among all answer choices you have not eliminated.

Copyright © Mometrix Media. You have been licensed one copy of this document for personal use only. Any other reproduction or redistribution is strictly prohibited. All rights reserved.
This content is provided for test preparation purposes only and does not imply an endorsement by Mometrix of any particular political, scientific, or religious point of view.

Test-Taking Strategies

This section contains a list of test-taking strategies that you may find helpful as you work through the test. By taking what you know and applying logical thought, you can maximize your chances of answering any question correctly!

It is very important to realize that every question is different and every person is different: no single strategy will work on every question, and no single strategy will work for every person. That's why we've included all of them here, so you can try them out and determine which ones work best for different types of questions and which ones work best for you.

Question Strategies

⊘ Read Carefully

Read the question and the answer choices carefully. Don't miss the question because you misread the terms. You have plenty of time to read each question thoroughly and make sure you understand what is being asked. Yet a happy medium must be attained, so don't waste too much time. You must read carefully and efficiently.

⊘ Contextual Clues

Look for contextual clues. If the question includes a word you are not familiar with, look at the immediate context for some indication of what the word might mean. Contextual clues can often give you all the information you need to decipher the meaning of an unfamiliar word. Even if you can't determine the meaning, you may be able to narrow down the possibilities enough to make a solid guess at the answer to the question.

⊘ Prefixes

If you're having trouble with a word in the question or answer choices, try dissecting it. Take advantage of every clue that the word might include. Prefixes can be a huge help. Usually, they allow you to determine a basic meaning. *Pre-* means before, *post-* means after, *pro-* is positive, *de-* is negative. From prefixes, you can get an idea of the general meaning of the word and try to put it into context.

⊘ Hedge Words

Watch out for critical hedge words, such as *likely, may, can, often, almost, mostly, usually, generally, rarely,* and *sometimes.* Question writers insert these hedge phrases to cover every possibility. Often an answer choice will be wrong simply because it leaves no room for exception. Be on guard for answer choices that have definitive words such as *exactly* and *always.*

Copyright © Mometrix Media. You have been licensed one copy of this document for personal use only. Any other reproduction or redistribution is strictly prohibited. All rights reserved.
This content is provided for test preparation purposes only and does not imply an endorsement by Mometrix of any particular political, scientific, or religious point of view.

⊘ Switchback Words

Stay alert for *switchbacks*. These are the words and phrases frequently used to alert you to shifts in thought. The most common switchback words are *but*, *although*, and *however*. Others include *nevertheless*, *on the other hand*, *even though*, *while*, *in spite of*, *despite*, and *regardless of*. Switchback words are important to catch because they can change the direction of the question or an answer choice.

⊘ Face Value

When in doubt, use common sense. Accept the situation in the problem at face value. Don't read too much into it. These problems will not require you to make wild assumptions. If you have to go beyond creativity and warp time or space in order to have an answer choice fit the question, then you should move on and consider the other answer choices. These are normal problems rooted in reality. The applicable relationship or explanation may not be readily apparent, but it is there for you to figure out. Use your common sense to interpret anything that isn't clear.

Answer Choice Strategies

⊘ Answer Selection

The most thorough way to pick an answer choice is to identify and eliminate wrong answers until only one is left, then confirm it is the correct answer. Sometimes an answer choice may immediately seem right, but be careful. The test writers will usually put more than one reasonable answer choice on each question, so take a second to read all of them and make sure that the other choices are not equally obvious. As long as you have time left, it is better to read every answer choice than to pick the first one that looks right without checking the others.

⊘ Answer Choice Families

An answer choice family consists of two (in rare cases, three) answer choices that are very similar in construction and cannot all be true at the same time. If you see two answer choices that are direct opposites or parallels, one of them is usually the correct answer. For instance, if one answer choice says that quantity *x* increases and another either says that quantity *x* decreases (opposite) or says that quantity *y* increases (parallel), then those answer choices would fall into the same family. An answer choice that doesn't match the construction of the answer choice family is more likely to be incorrect. Most questions will not have answer choice families, but when they do appear, you should be prepared to recognize them.

⊘ Eliminate Answers

Eliminate answer choices as soon as you realize they are wrong, but make sure you consider all possibilities. If you are eliminating answer choices and realize that the last one you are left with is also wrong, don't panic. Start over and consider each choice again. There may be something you missed the first time that you will realize on the second pass.

Copyright © Mometrix Media. You have been licensed one copy of this document for personal use only. Any other reproduction or redistribution is strictly prohibited. All rights reserved.
This content is provided for test preparation purposes only and does not imply an endorsement by Mometrix of any particular political, scientific, or religious point of view.

✓ AVOID FACT TRAPS

Don't be distracted by an answer choice that is factually true but doesn't answer the question. You are looking for the choice that answers the question. Stay focused on what the question is asking for so you don't accidentally pick an answer that is true but incorrect. Always go back to the question and make sure the answer choice you've selected actually answers the question and is not merely a true statement.

✓ EXTREME STATEMENTS

In general, you should avoid answers that put forth extreme actions as standard practice or proclaim controversial ideas as established fact. An answer choice that states the "process should be used in certain situations, if..." is much more likely to be correct than one that states the "process should be discontinued completely." The first is a calm rational statement and doesn't even make a definitive, uncompromising stance, using a hedge word *if* to provide wiggle room, whereas the second choice is far more extreme.

✓ BENCHMARK

As you read through the answer choices and you come across one that seems to answer the question well, mentally select that answer choice. This is not your final answer, but it's the one that will help you evaluate the other answer choices. The one that you selected is your benchmark or standard for judging each of the other answer choices. Every other answer choice must be compared to your benchmark. That choice is correct until proven otherwise by another answer choice beating it. If you find a better answer, then that one becomes your new benchmark. Once you've decided that no other choice answers the question as well as your benchmark, you have your final answer.

✓ PREDICT THE ANSWER

Before you even start looking at the answer choices, it is often best to try to predict the answer. When you come up with the answer on your own, it is easier to avoid distractions and traps because you will know exactly what to look for. The right answer choice is unlikely to be word-for-word what you came up with, but it should be a close match. Even if you are confident that you have the right answer, you should still take the time to read each option before moving on.

General Strategies

✓ TOUGH QUESTIONS

If you are stumped on a problem or it appears too hard or too difficult, don't waste time. Move on! Remember though, if you can quickly check for obviously incorrect answer choices, your chances of guessing correctly are greatly improved. Before you completely give up, at least try to knock out a couple of possible answers. Eliminate what you can and then guess at the remaining answer choices before moving on.

Copyright © Mometrix Media. You have been licensed one copy of this document for personal use only. Any other reproduction or redistribution is strictly prohibited. All rights reserved.
This content is provided for test preparation purposes only and does not imply an endorsement by Mometrix of any particular political, scientific, or religious point of view.

⊘ Check Your Work

Since you will probably not know every term listed and the answer to every question, it is important that you get credit for the ones that you do know. Don't miss any questions through careless mistakes. If at all possible, try to take a second to look back over your answer selection and make sure you've selected the correct answer choice and haven't made a costly careless mistake (such as marking an answer choice that you didn't mean to mark). This quick double check should more than pay for itself in caught mistakes for the time it costs.

⊘ Pace Yourself

It's easy to be overwhelmed when you're looking at a page full of questions; your mind is confused and full of random thoughts, and the clock is ticking down faster than you would like. Calm down and maintain the pace that you have set for yourself. Especially as you get down to the last few minutes of the test, don't let the small numbers on the clock make you panic. As long as you are on track by monitoring your pace, you are guaranteed to have time for each question.

⊘ Don't Rush

It is very easy to make errors when you are in a hurry. Maintaining a fast pace in answering questions is pointless if it makes you miss questions that you would have gotten right otherwise. Test writers like to include distracting information and wrong answers that seem right. Taking a little extra time to avoid careless mistakes can make all the difference in your test score. Find a pace that allows you to be confident in the answers that you select.

⊘ Keep Moving

Panicking will not help you pass the test, so do your best to stay calm and keep moving. Taking deep breaths and going through the answer elimination steps you practiced can help to break through a stress barrier and keep your pace.

Copyright © Mometrix Media. You have been licensed one copy of this document for personal use only. Any other reproduction or redistribution is strictly prohibited. All rights reserved.
This content is provided for test preparation purposes only and does not imply an endorsement by Mometrix of any particular political, scientific, or religious point of view.

Final Notes

The combination of a solid foundation of content knowledge and the confidence that comes from practicing your plan for applying that knowledge is the key to maximizing your performance on test day. As your foundation of content knowledge is built up and strengthened, you'll find that the strategies included in this chapter become more and more effective in helping you quickly sift through the distractions and traps of the test to isolate the correct answer.

Now that you're preparing to move forward into the test content chapters of this book, be sure to keep your goal in mind. As you read, think about how you will be able to apply this information on the test. If you've already seen sample questions for the test and you have an idea of the question format and style, try to come up with questions of your own that you can answer based on what you're reading. This will give you valuable practice applying your knowledge in the same ways you can expect to on test day.

Good luck and good studying!

Copyright © Mometrix Media. You have been licensed one copy of this document for personal use only. Any other reproduction or redistribution is strictly prohibited. All rights reserved.
This content is provided for test preparation purposes only and does not imply an endorsement by Mometrix of any particular political, scientific, or religious point of view.

Copyright © Mometrix Media. You have been licensed one copy of this document for personal use only. Any other reproduction or redistribution is strictly prohibited. All rights reserved.
This content is provided for test preparation purposes only and does not imply an endorsement by Mometrix of any particular political, scientific, or religious point of view.

Normal Anatomy, Perfusion, and Function

Aortoiliac Vasculature

Blood Flow from the Heart to the Abdominal Aorta

Oxygenated blood leaves the heart and is pumped into the aorta, which contains several arterial branches to carry the blood to all cells of the body. The aorta has four major sections and is the longest artery in the human body. From the left ventricle of the heart, the blood is first pumped into a short segment of the aorta known as the ascending aorta. Next, the oxygenated blood reaches the aortic arch before it becomes the descending (thoracic) aorta. The fourth segment arises once this blood vessel passes through a small opening in the diaphragm. Here, it is known as the abdominal aorta. It is the largest artery in the abdominal cavity, and it supplies the organs and tissues of the abdomen, pelvis, and lower extremities with oxygenated blood.

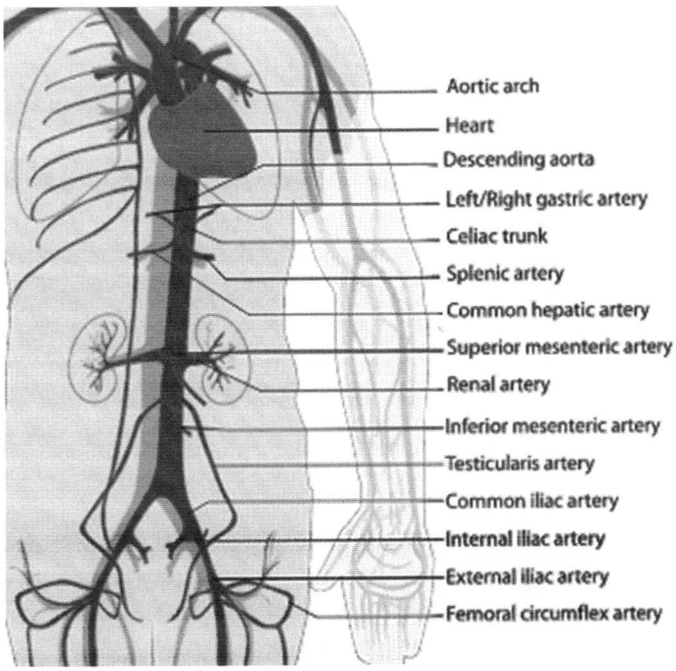

Blood Flow from the Distal Portion of the Abdominal Aorta

The thoracic aorta becomes the abdominal aorta once it passes through the diaphragm to carry oxygenated blood away from the heart. This artery eventually bifurcates at the level of the fourth lumbar vertebra to become the right and left common iliac arteries. These arteries extend to about the level of the last lumbar vertebra or proximal sacral region and eventually continue as the right and left external iliac arteries. These arteries descend to become the common femoral arteries as they descend inferior and laterally along the psoas muscle's medial margin. The external iliac arteries are referred as the right and left common femoral

Copyright © Mometrix Media. You have been licensed one copy of this document for personal use only. Any other reproduction or redistribution is strictly prohibited. All rights reserved.
This content is provided for test preparation purposes only and does not imply an endorsement by Mometrix of any particular political, scientific, or religious point of view.

arteries once they have continued past (beneath) the right and left inguinal ligament. Conversely, the internal iliac (also referred to as the hypogastric) arteries actually branch off of and course medially to the common iliac arteries to supply oxygenated blood to the wall of the external genitalia, buttocks, thigh, and wall of the pelvis.

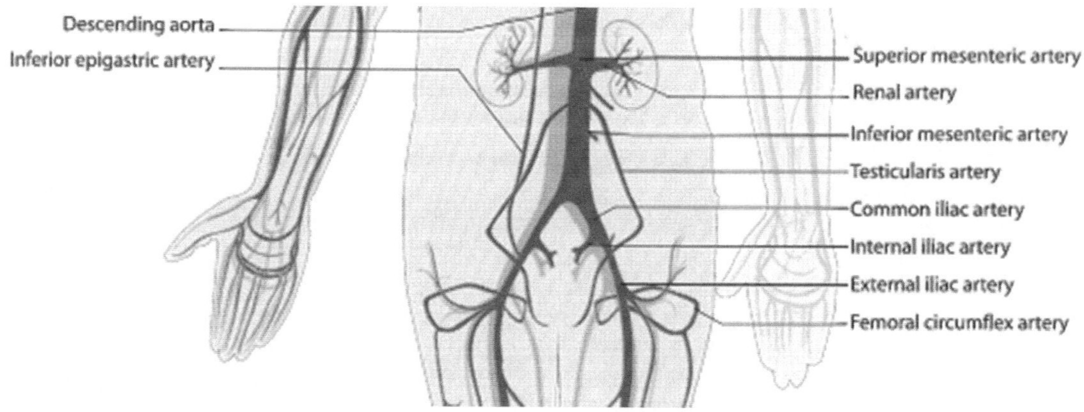

Superior Mesenteric Artery

The second main artery to branch from the abdominal aorta is the superior mesenteric artery (SMA). The origin of the SMA is roughly 1 cm from the point at which the first branch of the abdominal aorta stems from. This arterial trunk is named the celiac axis. However, in some patients the celiac artery and SMA may emerge from the same trunk. The SMA branches off the abdominal aorta anteriorly and then runs posterior to the pancreatic neck and splenic vein. Several important branches of the SMA supply oxygenated blood to the digestive system, especially those on the right side of the body. The cecum (which is the first portion of the colon) and ascending colon are on the right side of the patient's body and converge with the right half of the transverse colon and are all fed by the branches of the SMA.

Anomalies Affecting the Aortic Arch

Anomalies of the aortic arch are called congenital malformations because they are present at birth. The first branch of the aorta is the innominate (also referred to as the brachiocephalic) artery. The second artery to stem from the aortic arch is the left common carotid artery (CCA), with the left subclavian artery as the third division. Although there are multiple anatomical arrangements outside of the normal configurations, the most common variation occurs when the innominate and left common carotid arteries arise from the same region of the aortic arch. Sometimes, the left CCA will originate from the innominate artery (however, this is a less common scenario). Another anomaly of the aortic arch is the visualization of the left vertebral artery that originates directly from the arch in a more proximal location than the left subclavian artery instead of branching from the left subclavian artery.

Copyright © Mometrix Media. You have been licensed one copy of this document for personal use only. Any other reproduction or redistribution is strictly prohibited. All rights reserved.
This content is provided for test preparation purposes only and does not imply an endorsement by Mometrix of any particular political, scientific, or religious point of view.

Upper Extremity Veins

Superficial and Deep Veins

The deep venous system is a network of veins that acts as a conduit to return blood from the systemic circulatory system back to the heart. The deep veins usually have an artery that can be tracked parallel to the vein. The deep veins are often in a more internal location when compared to the superficial veins, which are found near the surface. The ulnar and radial veins are paired vessels (meaning there are two of them), are located near the ulnar artery and radial artery, and are considered deep veins. The axillary vein, brachial vein, and deep palmar venous arch are also part of the deep venous system. The cephalic and basilic veins are not joined by an artery with the same label and are not paired; instead, they are part of the superficial venous system. Note that the cephalic vein runs along the lateral portion of the arm, whereas the basilic vein is found on the medial aspect of the arm (remember the correct anatomical position).

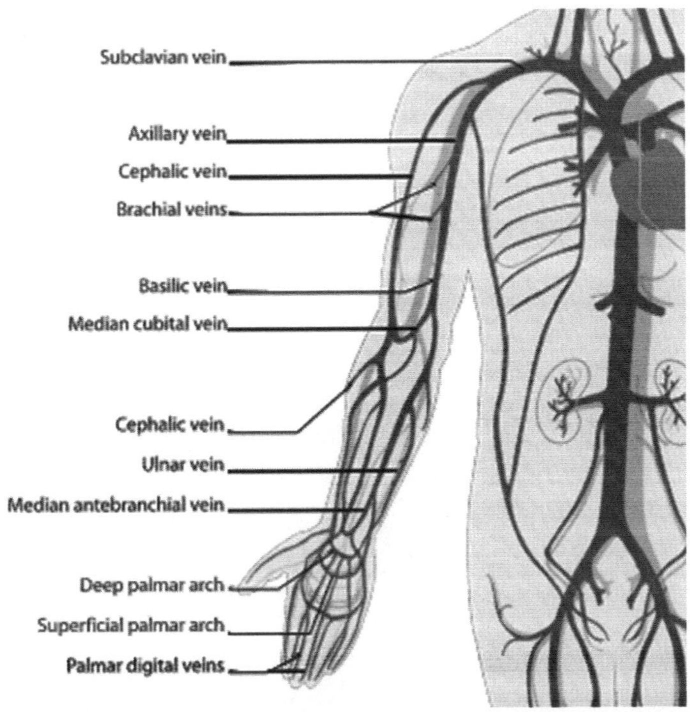

Pathway of Blood After It Reaches the Right and Left Innominate Veins

The right and left innominate veins, also known as the brachiocephalic veins, are formed by the confluence of the internal jugular vein in the neck and the subclavian vein. The right innominate vein receives blood from the right side of their body above the level of the heart to include the brain, neck, and right arm via the subclavian vein, whereas the left innominate vein receives blood from the left side of the body above the level of the heart to include the brain, neck, and left arm via the subclavian vein. The left innominate vein is longer than the right because it needs to reach the right atrium of the heart. The right and left innominate veins merge to form the superior vena cava (SVC). The SVC dumps deoxygenated blood into the right atrium of the heart.

Copyright © Mometrix Media. You have been licensed one copy of this document for personal use only. Any other reproduction or redistribution is strictly prohibited. All rights reserved.
This content is provided for test preparation purposes only and does not imply an endorsement by Mometrix of any particular political, scientific, or religious point of view.

Brachiocephalic Veins vs. the Brachiocephalic Artery

The venous system consists of bilateral brachiocephalic veins. The right and left brachiocephalic veins are also referred to as the right and left innominate veins, which allow the blood to flow from the internal jugular and subclavian veins on both sides of the body. Collectively, these vessels aid in returning blood that has been depleted of oxygen from regions superior to the heart back to the right atrium via the SVC when they merge. It is important to note that the arterial system varies, however, because there is only one brachiocephalic artery that stems from the aortic arch. This is also known as the innominate artery, and it supplies oxygenated blood to the right side of the neck, the head, as well as the right upper extremity. The innominate artery can supply these anatomical structures because it branches into the right carotid and subclavian arteries.

Avoiding Confusion Using Terminology

The veins carry blood that has been depleted of oxygen back to the heart. Because of the direction that blood travels within the veins, it is helpful to use terminology that will help avoid any confusion in regard to which segment of the vessel is being examined or discussed. Often, the terms proximal and distal are used, but it can often be helpful when evaluating the veins of the upper extremities to use the terms cranial and caudal instead. Transverse imaging is 90 degrees (or perpendicular) to the vein's long axis. The longitudinal imaging plane is parallel to the long axis of the blood vessel.

Lower Extremity Veins

Great Saphenous Vein

The longest vein in the body is the great saphenous vein (GSV), which is found in the medial surface of the legs. There is a right and left GSV, and these vessels start on the top of the foot and ascend anteriorly to the medial malleoli while continuing to the saphenofemoral junction (SFJ). The SFJ is where the GSV finally merges with the common femoral vein (CFV) in the patient's proximal thigh. The GSV does contain valves, and more of these structures are located inferior to the knee. The GSV can receive blood from the entire leg because of the various tributaries that drain blood into it. The GSV is known as a superficial vein not only because of its superficial

Copyright © Mometrix Media. You have been licensed one copy of this document for personal use only. Any other reproduction or redistribution is strictly prohibited. All rights reserved.
This content is provided for test preparation purposes only and does not imply an endorsement by Mometrix of any particular political, scientific, or religious point of view.

location, but because there is not an artery associated with it. The GSV is often harvested for use as a graft during coronary artery bypass surgery.

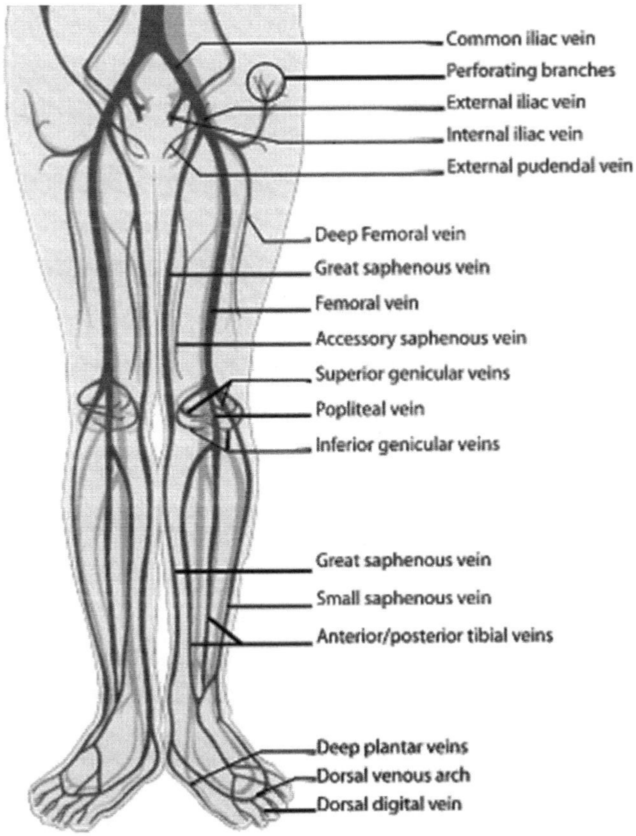

Major Veins in the Groin and Pelvis

The CFVs are found in the proximal portions of the thighs in the right and left lower extremities. As this vessel ascends into the groin, it becomes the external iliac vein at a level superior to the inguinal ligament. The common iliac vein is the result of the confluence of the internal iliac vein and the external iliac vein. The inferior vena cava (IVC) is the result of the right and left common iliac veins merging together in the abdomen typically at the level of the fifth lumbar vertebra. The IVC ascends in the abdomen just to the right of midline where it returns blood that has been depleted of oxygen to the right atrium of the heart.

Perforating and Communicating Veins

Perforating veins (also referred to as perforators) can be thought of as the vessels that join the superficial venous system to the deep veins. In fact, the pathway of blood draining from the lower limbs passes through the superficial veins into the perforators and then moves into the deep venous system. These veins are typically located within the muscle and are associated with a perforating artery. These vessels contain valves to ensure one-way blood flow to help blood reach the deep system such as those in the thigh and lower leg. Notably, the perforators located in the foot move blood into the superficial system instead of the deep system. There are also vessels known as communicating veins, which allow blood to travel in the

Copyright © Mometrix Media. You have been licensed one copy of this document for personal use only. Any other reproduction or redistribution is strictly prohibited. All rights reserved.
This content is provided for test preparation purposes only and does not imply an endorsement by Mometrix of any particular political, scientific, or religious point of view.

same venous systems, for example, from the superficial venous system to superficial veins or from the deep venous system to deep veins. These are typically very small (less than 2 mm) and cannot typically be seen during a venous duplex ultrasound.

Difficulty Visualizing the Femoral Vein

During a venous duplex exam, the femoral vein is often difficult to visualize well in the distal thigh because it tends to run deeper in the lower third of the leg when compared to the mid and proximal thigh as it is approached from the popliteal region. The popliteal vein advances through an area known as the adductor hiatus (also referred to as Hunter's canal). This area contains an opening that allows the passage of the popliteal vein to course from the posterior portion of the knee to the anterior thigh. In the distal thigh, the vascular technologist may find it helpful to interrogate the distal femoral vein on the posterior surface instead of from a more medial or anterior approach.

Gastrocnemius and Soleal Veins

In order to assist in the blood return from the lower extremities to the heart, the gastrocnemius and soleal muscles must act as a muscle pump (with the soleal sinuses acting as the main supply). The contractions in the calf and ankle region aid in blood return by forcing the blood that is in the veins to move toward the heart when walking or performing any motion that flexes the foot. It is important to note that the gastrocnemius and soleal veins can develop blood clots; these may be seen during lower venous duplex exams. There are typically multiple gastrocnemius veins found in the calf region that drain directly into the popliteal vein of the lower leg. These vessels contain functioning valves. Deep vein thromboses (DVTs) that develop in the soleal veins are believed to be responsible for a large percentage of pulmonary emboli. The soleal sinuses tend to drain into the peroneal and posterior tibial veins.

Normal Peripheral Venous vs. Arterial Waveforms

The venous system returns oxygen back to the right atrium of the heart. The blood from the lower extremities returns to the heart via the IVC. The pressure within the venous system is much lower than the pressure found in the arterial system, and when interrogating peripheral veins above the knee with spectral Doppler, it should demonstrate spontaneous flow. Spontaneous blood flow confirms that the vessel is not obstructed. The venous waveform should be phasic when the patient inhales and exhales. The blood in the arterial system is transferred out of the heart and delivered to all of the body's cells. The spectral waveform of the peripheral arteries will typically exhibit blood flow that has high resistance and is either biphasic or triphasic with bidirectional flow. If a patient presents with narrowing of the arteries, the waveform tends to demonstrate continuous flow in only one direction with decreased resistance.

Protocol and Sonographic Findings When Negative for a DVT

The venous system is a network of veins that returns blood that has been depleted of oxygen back to the right atrium of the heart. The vessel walls of veins and arteries

Copyright © Mometrix Media. You have been licensed one copy of this document for personal use only. Any other reproduction or redistribution is strictly prohibited. All rights reserved.
This content is provided for test preparation purposes only and does not imply an endorsement by Mometrix of any particular political, scientific, or religious point of view.

consist of three separate layers, but the layers in veins tend to be thinner, which allows the vessel to be compressed during a venous duplex exam. A venous duplex exam is performed to diagnose the presence of a deep vein thrombosis (DVT). The protocol includes gray-scale, color, and spectral Doppler starting at the groin in the transverse plane compressing the veins with light pressure from the transducer. A vein that can be compressed wall to wall does not contain a clot (which can usually be seen with gray-scale and color Doppler). Nonobstructed veins above the knee should demonstrate spontaneous flow and phasicity with changes in respiration. Some labs also use augmentation to show that there isn't a clot between the calf and a more proximal location that is being scanned.

Effect of Breathing on Blood Flow

When a spectral analysis of blood flow of the legs is performed in a patient that has patent veins, the signal will demonstrate phasic flow when the patient is breathing. In the lower extremities, the signal decreases upon inhalation and increases when the patient exhales. When the patient inhales, there is increased intra-abdominal pressure, which, in turn, lessens the flow from the legs. Upon exhalation, there is decreased intra-abdominal pressure, which enables the blood flow from the legs to increase. Vascular technologists should be aware that the opposite is true when assessing the upper extremities because the signal increases with inhalation and decreases when the patient exhales. When the Valsalva maneuver is performed, pressure in the thoracic and abdominal cavities rises, which creates a cessation of flow to the heart that interrupts all blood flow in the body.

Native Upper Extremity Arteries

Blood Flow After It Reaches the Brachial Artery

The brachial artery is found in the upper arm and is used to determine an individual's blood pressure. The brachial artery receives blood flow from the axillary artery and carries it to the antecubital fossa, which is located in the anterior region of the arm where the elbow bends. It is in this region that the brachial artery branches into the radial and ulnar arteries. The radial artery is found on the same side as one of the bones of the forearm known as the radius (located on the lateral or thumb side). The ulnar artery is the other branch that stems from the brachial artery and is found on the medial (pinkie) side of the forearm. The radial and ulnar arteries supply the hand with the necessary blood flow.

Spectral Waveform Seen in a Normal Brachial Artery

When a vascular technologist is interrogating the arteries of the upper extremities with spectral Doppler, it is important to note that the waveform of the brachial artery should display high resistance. This is because it is a peripheral artery with smaller distal arterioles that impedes the blood flow from arteries to the more distal arterioles. Depending on the age of the patient, normal waveforms of the brachial artery will demonstrate a triphasic or biphasic waveform. As people age, elasticity is lost in the blood vessels, which can result in a more biphasic flow. In younger individuals, a short reversal of flow will be demonstrated at the end of systole and

Copyright © Mometrix Media. You have been licensed one copy of this document for personal use only. Any other reproduction or redistribution is strictly prohibited. All rights reserved.
This content is provided for test preparation purposes only and does not imply an endorsement by Mometrix of any particular political, scientific, or religious point of view.

then the blood flows forward once again. This triphasic waveform also demonstrates a brisk upstroke and downstroke during systole.

Origin of the Subclavian Arteries

There are two subclavian arteries (one on each side of the body), and it is important to note that the origins of the right and left subclavian arteries are very different. The right subclavian artery is the result of the bifurcation of the innominate (brachiocephalic) artery, which is the first division of the aortic arch that originates from the right side. The innominate artery bifurcates and branches into the right CCA as well as the right subclavian artery. The left subclavian artery stems from the arch of the aorta and is the third vessel to stem from the arch. The subclavian arteries give off several branches with the vertebral artery being one of the arteries that vascular technologists will interrogate during carotid duplex exams. The subclavian arteries are found just above the clavicles and becomes the axillary artery upon reaching the ribs.

Native Lower Extremity Arteries

Hunter's Canal

The area known as Hunter's canal is an important region located near the knee because it serves as a tunnel that allows the blood vessels of the thigh and lower leg to pass through the region of the popliteal fossa. For example, the femoral artery enters the posterior area of the knee to become the popliteal artery. The popliteal vein also passes through this region to become the femoral vein in the distal thigh. Often, the distal femoral vein cannot be seen due the depth of the vein in the area of Hunter's canal, so it may be necessary to scan from a more posterior approach. Another name for Hunter's canal is the adductor canal.

Blood Flow from the Popliteal Artery

The femoral artery of the thigh extends through an area known as the adductor (Hunter's) canal and becomes the popliteal artery in the region of the posterior knee. The popliteal artery is a relatively short blood vessel that supplies oxygenated blood to the knee and surrounding tissues. Although this blood vessel tends to be very short, it does have branches to supply the skin and muscles, which can serve as collateral vessels in cases of obstruction. The first vessel to stem from the popliteal artery is the anterior tibial artery, which supplies oxygenated blood to the lower leg and foot. The popliteal artery also branches into the tibioperoneal trunk, which gives off several branches to also supply blood to the lower leg and foot.

Popliteal Trifurcation

The area of the lower extremity known as the popliteal trifurcation is where the anterior tibial artery and the tibioperoneal trunk branch from the peroneal artery in the posterior region of the knee. This is an important area to evaluate because it is a common site for atherosclerosis to develop. The anterior tibial artery is the first artery to stem from the popliteal artery, and it courses along the anterior (front) of the lower leg to become the dorsalis pedis artery (DPA). The tibioperoneal trunk is the second arterial segment to divide from the peroneal artery. This trunk bifurcates

Copyright © Mometrix Media. You have been licensed one copy of this document for personal use only. Any other reproduction or redistribution is strictly prohibited. All rights reserved.
This content is provided for test preparation purposes only and does not imply an endorsement by Mometrix of any particular political, scientific, or religious point of view.

to form the peroneal artery, which supplies blood to the lateral region of the lower leg as well as the posterior tibial artery (PTA). The PTA runs along the medial side of the leg to carry blood to the foot.

Blood Flow from the External Iliac Artery

Recall that the arterial system carries oxygenated blood from the heart. As the blood flows away from the heart and into the abdominal aorta bifurcation, it is directed toward the right and left common iliac arteries at the level of the fourth lumbar vertebra. This bifurcation enables these vessels to carry blood to the pelvis via the internal iliac (hypogastric) artery and lower extremities via the external iliac arteries. The external iliac artery is the result of another bifurcation of the common iliac artery as it branches into the internal and external iliac arteries. The external iliac artery continues down the leg to become the common femoral artery (CFA) once it travels under the inguinal ligament. The CFA continues down the thigh and becomes the femoral artery to eventually become the popliteal artery once it reaches the posterior region of the knee.

Effect of Exercise on Peripheral Arteries

Peripheral resistance is a common term that is discussed in vascular ultrasound. As arteries extend in a more distal location, they typically become smaller in diameter as they approach the terminal arterioles. This decrease in the diameter of the blood vessels increases the resistance of blood that is moving within the peripheral arteries. Exercise will enable vasodilation within the smaller vessels, which will decrease the amount of peripheral resistance so that more blood can reach the skeletal muscles, which is a requirement during exercise. Flow reversal in a spectral Doppler waveform will be decreased, and the signal becomes one that demonstrates low resistance during exercise.

Mesenteric Vasculature

Celiac Trunk and Its Branches

The celiac trunk (also referred to as the celiac axis) is found in the abdomen and supplies blood to various digestive organs. The celiac trunk originates from the anterior surface of the abdominal aorta as the first branch. The celiac trunk is a short segment that gives off three main branches, which are the splenic, left gastric, and common hepatic arteries. The splenic artery supplies blood to the spleen, stomach, and the pancreas. The left gastric artery supplies blood to the stomach and

Copyright © Mometrix Media. You have been licensed one copy of this document for personal use only. Any other reproduction or redistribution is strictly prohibited. All rights reserved.
This content is provided for test preparation purposes only and does not imply an endorsement by Mometrix of any particular political, scientific, or religious point of view.

esophagus. The common hepatic artery supplies blood to the liver as well as the gallbladder.

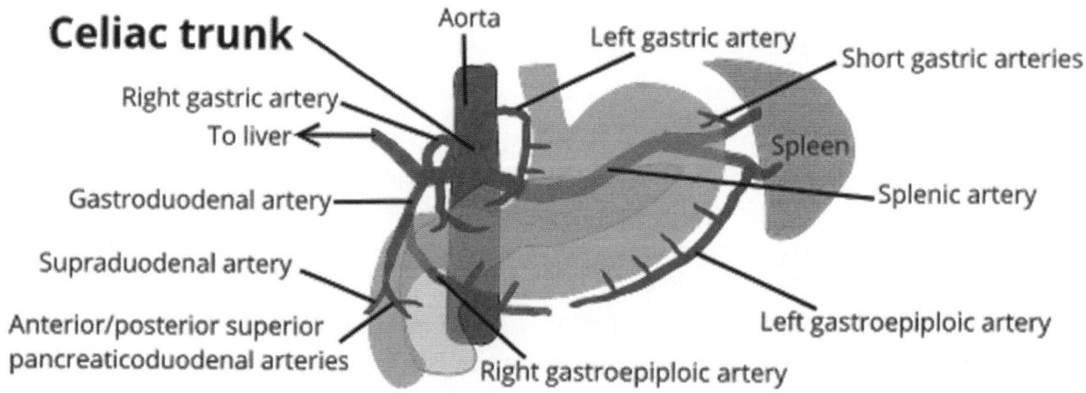

Perfusion of Normal Mesenteric Arteries

Vascular technologists should be aware that blood flow in the SMA is vastly different in fasting and postprandial states. When the patient has been fasting, the SMA should display a high-resistance waveform with flow reversal. The postprandial spectral Doppler waveform should demonstrate more blood flow in order to aid in digestion and will therefore have a higher peak-systolic velocity (PSV) and end-diastolic velocity (EDV). This increase in flow is the result of the vasodilation of arteries that supply oxygenated blood to the organs of digestion. The waveform of the celiac artery will not be altered when scanned after the patient eats. Some protocols include having the patient drink a high-caloric drink especially if he or she has a mesenteric bypass graft to compare the blood flow before and after eating.

Renal Vasculature

Challenges in Identifying the Renal Arteries

Visualization of the renal arteries is often technically challenging due to bowel gas that can obstruct the image. The patient should fast prior to this exam to decrease the amount of bowel gas that will obscure the renal arteries. The vascular technologist should use a 3–5 MHz curvilinear transducer to help penetrate the patient's abdomen. The origin of the renal arteries is slightly distal to where the SMA branches from the abdominal aorta. Many vascular labs require the kidneys as well as the abdominal aorta to be examined as part of a renal artery Doppler exam. If the origins of the renal arteries are not well visualized from the anterior approach, it may be useful to turn the patient on his or her left side to use a coronal approach for what is known as the "banana peel" sign to locate the origins of the right and left renal arteries. Color Doppler is recommended to help the technologist locate these vessels.

Purpose and Length of the Renal Veins

The purpose of the renal veins is to carry blood that has been depleted of oxygen back to the heart. These vessels drain into the IVC so that the blood can be returned to the right atrium. Recall that the IVC is situated to the right of the body, so the left renal vein is longer because it must extend across the midline of the body in order to

Copyright © Mometrix Media. You have been licensed one copy of this document for personal use only. Any other reproduction or redistribution is strictly prohibited. All rights reserved.
This content is provided for test preparation purposes only and does not imply an endorsement by Mometrix of any particular political, scientific, or religious point of view.

reach the IVC. In fact, the left renal vein crosses in front of the abdominal aorta but underneath one of the anterior branches of the abdominal aorta known as the SMA. The right renal vein tends to be shorter because the IVC is already just to the right of midline, so it is a much shorter distance to the IVC.

Blood Flow from the Renal Hilum to the Renal Cortex

The renal arteries supply oxygenated blood traveling from the abdominal aorta to the adrenal glands, ureters, as well as the kidneys. Once the main renal artery enters the renal hilum, it branches into five segmental arteries that supply the various regions of the kidney. As these vessels travel further outward to the periphery of the kidney, they branch to become the interlobar arteries. These arteries are found near the renal pyramids. The arcuate arteries tend to curve around the base of the renal pyramids to finally supply blood to the renal cortex. These arteries are known as the interlobular arteries. Blood flow from the renal hilum to the cortex is as follows:

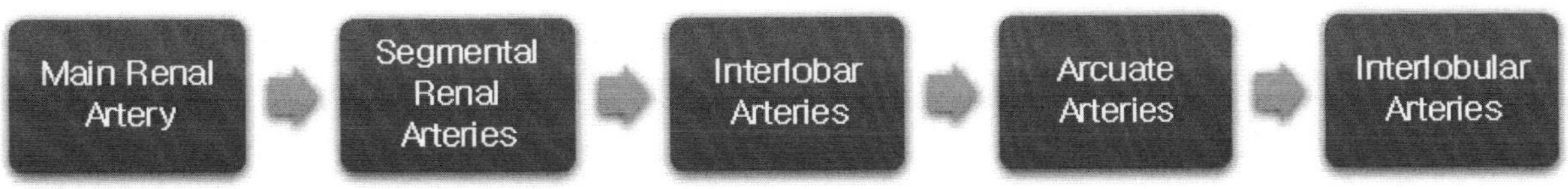
Main Renal Artery
Segmental Renal Arteries
Interlobar Arteries
Arcuate Arteries
Interlobular Arteries

Performing a Renal Arterial Duplex Exam

Many labs require the vascular technologist to image the abdominal aorta as well as the kidneys to assess the size and to look for any pathology that may be present. Typically, the blood flow in the renal arteries is seen as being of low resistance, while the aortic flow is of high resistance. In the proximal, mid, and distal segments of the renal arteries, the peak systolic and end-diastolic velocities are measured bilaterally. The peak systolic and end-diastolic velocities should also be sampled in the upper and lower poles within the segmental arteries and possibly the interlobar arteries. The renal-to-aortic ratio is calculated, and normal values will fall below 3.5. If the renal-to-aortic ratio is greater than or equal to 3.5, this suggests that a significant stenosis is present. The renal-to-aortic ratio is calculated by dividing the greatest peak-systolic velocity (PSV) of the renal artery by the greatest PSV of the abdominal aorta.

Position of the Left Renal Vein and the Abdominal Aorta

The right and left renal veins carry deoxygenated blood away from the kidneys into the IVC to be returned to the heart. The IVC is situated to the right of the midline in the abdomen, so the left renal vein must travel a greater distance than the right renal vein to return the blood into the IVC. The abdominal aorta is just to the left of the midline, which means that the left renal vein must cross anterior to the abdominal aorta before reaching the IVC. In a transverse plane, the left renal vein is seen between the SMA and the abdominal aorta, which may be another way to

Copyright © Mometrix Media. You have been licensed one copy of this document for personal use only. Any other reproduction or redistribution is strictly prohibited. All rights reserved.
This content is provided for test preparation purposes only and does not imply an endorsement by Mometrix of any particular political, scientific, or religious point of view.

locate the left renal artery during a Doppler exam because it is anterior to the left renal artery.

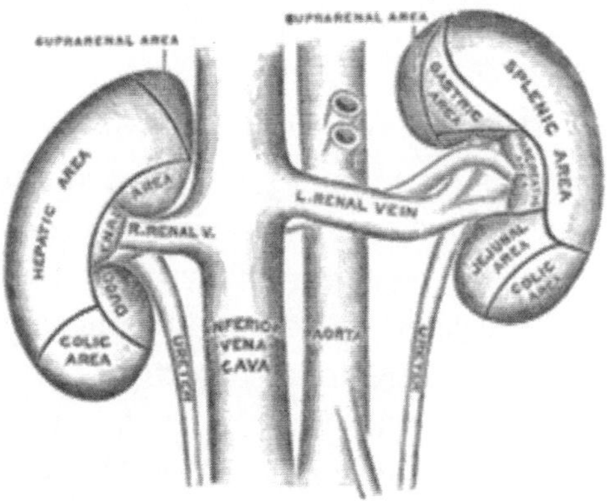

HEPATOPORTAL SYSTEM

PORTAL VEIN AND ITS BRANCHES

The main portal vein materializes from the confluence of several important vessels. These blood vessels drain the spleen and the intestines to transport blood to the liver in order to clear the blood of toxic materials. The splenic vein originates at the splenic hilum and passes posterior to the pancreatic tail and body until it reaches the head of the pancreas. Before the splenic vein reaches the head of the pancreas, it is joined by the inferior mesenteric vein. The landmark of the portal splenic confluence is found at the head of the pancreas where the splenic vein joins with the superior mesenteric vein. At the porta hepatis, this confluence emerges as the main portal vein , which divides into the left and right portal veins after it enters the liver. The left portal vein further divides into the lateral and medial branches within the

Copyright © Mometrix Media. You have been licensed one copy of this document for personal use only. Any other reproduction or redistribution is strictly prohibited. All rights reserved.
This content is provided for test preparation purposes only and does not imply an endorsement by Mometrix of any particular political, scientific, or religious point of view.

left lobe of the liver. Once it reaches the right lobe of the liver, the right portal vein branches into anterior and posterior divisions.

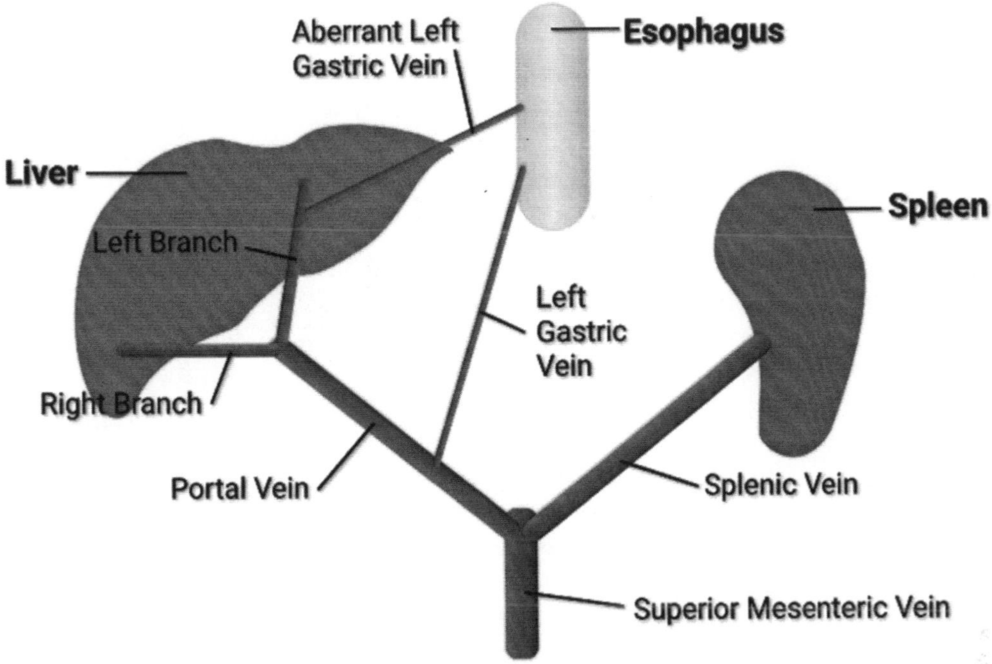

Hepatic Arterial vs. Portal Blood Flow to the Liver

Blood reaches the liver from two pathways: the hepatic arterial system and the portal system. The hepatic artery is a branch of the celiac artery, which is the first branch of the abdominal aorta. Although the hepatic artery supplies the majority of the oxygenated blood that the liver receives, it is actually only responsible for transporting about 25%–30% of the total blood volume into the liver. The rest of the blood volume (70%–75%) is transported to the liver from the main portal vein. Most of the blood that the portal vein transports has been depleted of oxygen and is traveling from the intestines to the liver to be cleaned. Portal veins tend to have a bright wall in a normal liver, whereas the hepatic arteries do not have echogenic walls. After the blood circulates through the liver, it is returned to the IVC from the hepatic veins.

Hepatopetal Blood Flow

The portal veins carry blood from the intestines into the liver in order to remove any toxic substances before it is returned to the heart. Normal flow in the portal veins will demonstrate hepatopetal flow, which means that the flow is moving toward the liver. If the blood flow is traveling away from the liver, it is known as hepatofugal flow. There are several reasons that a patient may experience reduced hepatopetal flow, and some of the main causes are portal hypertension (PHTN), cirrhosis, a blood clot, or tumor formation as seen in hepatocellular carcinoma. Typically, the blood flow within the portal vein may be somewhat pulsatile, but it is continuous with small respiratory variations as the patient breathes in and out (phasicity).

Copyright © Mometrix Media. You have been licensed one copy of this document for personal use only. Any other reproduction or redistribution is strictly prohibited. All rights reserved.
This content is provided for test preparation purposes only and does not imply an endorsement by Mometrix of any particular political, scientific, or religious point of view.

Inferior Vena Cava and/or Iliac Veins

Inferior Vena Cava and the Abdominal Aorta

The inferior vena cava (IVC) is a large vein that returns blood that has been depleted of oxygen back to the right atrium of the heart. The blood that is emptied into the IVC is from the level below the heart. The IVC sits to the right of the spine and is formed by the confluence of the common iliac veins. This confluence is usually found at the level of the fifth lumbar vertebra. The abdominal aorta carries oxygenated blood and is a continuance of the thoracic aorta once it passes through the diaphragm and sits to the left side of the spine. At the level of the fourth lumbar vertebra, the abdominal aorta bifurcates into the right and left common iliac arteries, which continue down each lower extremity. The distal portion of the abdominal aorta tends to sit anterior to the IVC; therefore, the right common iliac arteries are found in front of the common iliac veins. The aortic bifurcation is proximal to the location in which the common iliac veins merge to form the IVC.

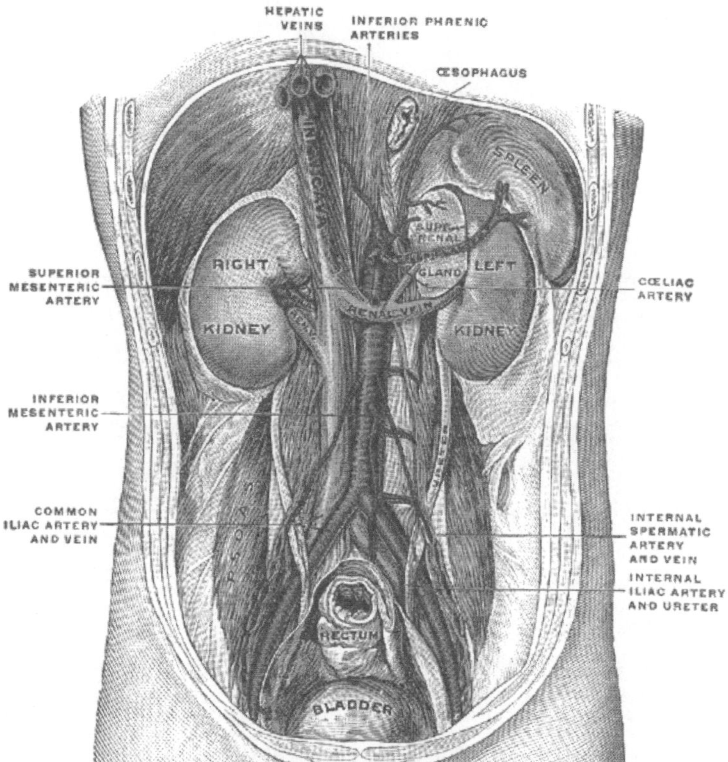

Inguinal Ligament as a Landmark for Vascular Imaging

The femoral triangle is an important anatomical region that physicians use when the femoral vein or artery needs to be used as an access point. The femoral triangle is located at the anterior portion of the thigh, and the inguinal ligament marks the superior-most border of the femoral triangle. The inguinal ligament is a structure that separates the thigh from the wall of the abdominal cavity. The inguinal ligament may be palpated by physicians in patients who are thin when vascular access is

Copyright © Mometrix Media. You have been licensed one copy of this document for personal use only. Any other reproduction or redistribution is strictly prohibited. All rights reserved.
This content is provided for test preparation purposes only and does not imply an endorsement by Mometrix of any particular political, scientific, or religious point of view.

necessary. Vascular technologists should use the inguinal ligament as a landmark to discern the external iliac artery from the common femoral artery (CFA) because this vessel becomes the CFA once it travels past and underneath it. The common femoral vein (CFV) is formed within the femoral triangle when the deep femoral vein (DFV) meets the superficial femoral vein (SFV). The CFV is found just medial to the CFA. The great saphenous vein (GSV) enters the CFV before it passes underneath the inguinal ligament, which then gives way to the vessel known as the external iliac vein.

Extracranial Cerebrovascular System

Innominate Artery

The ascending aorta becomes the aortic arch, which contains three major branches. The aortic arch is named as such because it curves up toward the back and then bends left prior to its plunge as the descending aorta. The first or most proximal branch that stems from the aortic arch is the innominate artery. This vessel is also known as the brachiocephalic artery or is even referenced as the brachiocephalic trunk of the aorta. This vessel is the branch that is the largest of the three branches of the aortic arch, and it supplies the right side of the brain, face, neck, and arm with oxygenated blood. The innominate artery gives rise to the right CCA and the right subclavian artery. Notably, the innominate artery is only found on the right side of the body.

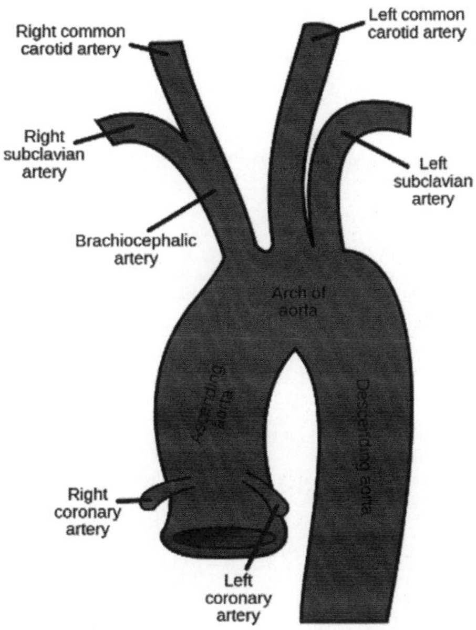

Left CCA and the Left Subclavian Artery

The aortic arch contains three significant branches. The left CCA supplies oxygenated blood to the left side of the brain, face, and neck and is the second branch of the aortic arch. Vascular technologists can follow the left CCA from the bottom of the neck in a cephalad direction to the carotid bifurcation. The right CCA, on the other hand, does not branch directly from the aortic arch, but rather from the innominate artery, which is the first vessel to branch from the arch. The left

Copyright © Mometrix Media. You have been licensed one copy of this document for personal use only. Any other reproduction or redistribution is strictly prohibited. All rights reserved.
This content is provided for test preparation purposes only and does not imply an endorsement by Mometrix of any particular political, scientific, or religious point of view.

subclavian artery is the third branch of the arch. This vessel carries oxygenated blood to the left upper extremity and branches several times to also supply blood to the chest. From the aortic arch, it passes above the clavicle to the lateral portion of the first rib to become the axillary artery.

Internal Thoracic Artery May Require Mapping

The subclavian artery has several branches, one of which is the internal thoracic artery. This artery is also referred to as the internal mammary artery, and it arises near the origin of the subclavian artery to descend along both sides of the sternum to supply oxygenated blood to the breasts and anterior wall of the thoracic cavity. This artery is often used by plastic surgeons in patients that have had a mastectomy as a microvascular anastomosis for transverse rectus abdominis myocutaneous flaps when patients have chosen to undergo breast reconstruction. Ultrasound can be used to determine patency and the size of the artery. The diameter of this artery should be 2 mm and should demonstrate low-resistance flow. Cardiothoracic surgeons may also use the internal thoracic artery when a coronary artery bypass surgery is necessary. The internal thoracic artery is often chosen because this type of graft has less risk of becoming occluded than grafts created by veins. The left internal thoracic artery is often used because of the close proximity to the heart.

Superior Thyroid Artery

The superior thyroid artery is a blood vessel that, as the name implies, is responsible for carrying oxygenated blood to the thyroid gland. The thyroid gland is a butterfly-shaped gland situated at the base of the neck near the midline. Its location explains why the direction of blood flow in the superior thyroid arterial branch moves in the opposite direction when compared to normal carotid arteries as it is moving inferior to the bottom of the neck. Vascular technologists can typically see the superior thyroid artery when performing a carotid duplex study because it is the first of eight branches of the external carotid artery (ECA). On occasion, the superior thyroid artery may arise from the distal segment of the CCA. The superior thyroid artery has several arterial branches to supply neighboring tissues.

Ophthalmic Artery

The internal carotid artery (ICA) originates at the bifurcation of the CCA in the neck. The ICA has several branches to carry oxygenated blood to the brain and eyes. Typically, during a carotid duplex ultrasound, the divisions of the ICA are not seen because the divisions are not extracranial (recall that the branches of the ECA, however, can be seen in the neck). The first major intracranial division of the ICA is the ophthalmic artery, which supplies the eye with oxygenated blood. The ophthalmic artery is often seen at the curve of the ICA known as the carotid siphon, and it has several branches that supply various parts of the eye, the muscles that move the eyeball, as well as the eyelid. Notably, some of the arteries that stem from the ophthalmic artery connect with some of the ECA branches and may act as collateral channels if the ICA is diseased.

Copyright © Mometrix Media. You have been licensed one copy of this document for personal use only. Any other reproduction or redistribution is strictly prohibited. All rights reserved.
This content is provided for test preparation purposes only and does not imply an endorsement by Mometrix of any particular political, scientific, or religious point of view.

VERTEBRAL ARTERIES

The right and left subclavian arteries serve as the origin of the right and left vertebral arteries. The vertebral arteries travel superiorly in the neck as the first division of the subclavian arteries in a more posterior position than the ICA. In fact, starting with the foramen of the sixth cervical (C6) vertebra, the vertebral arteries continue to pass through the foramina of the more superior cervical vertebrae to travel upward toward the base of the skull to enter the foramen magnum, which is found in the posterior portion of the skull. The foramen magnum is a large opening in the occipital bone that allows the brain stem and spinal cord to unite. These arteries join to form the basilar artery, which supplies oxygenated blood to the posterior structures of the brain. The vertebral arteries are not typically the same size because the left vertebral artery is often slightly larger than the right.

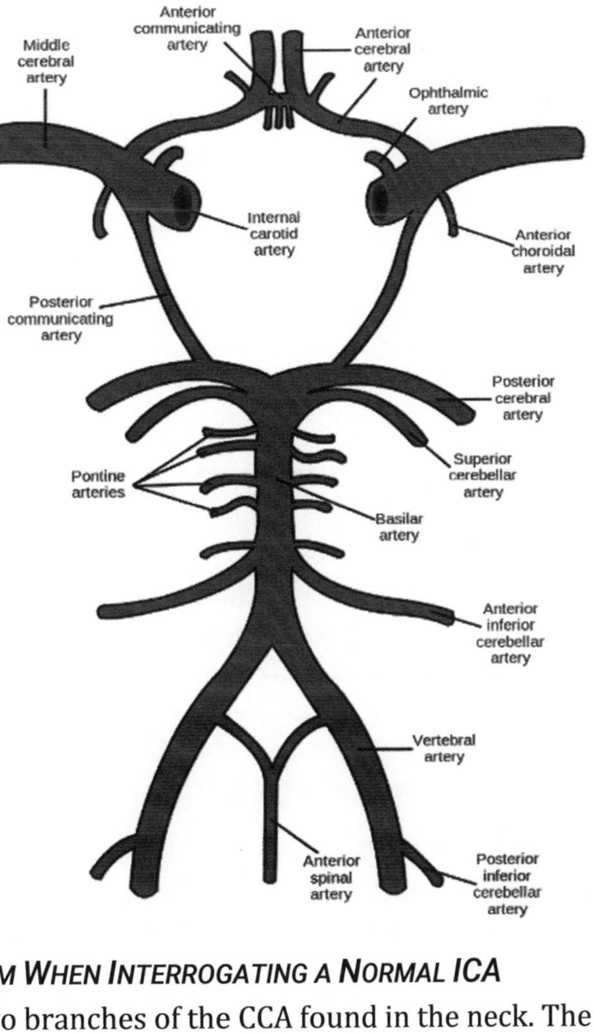

SPECTRAL WAVEFORM WHEN INTERROGATING A NORMAL ICA

The ICA is one of two branches of the CCA found in the neck. The ICA is the blood vessel that transports the majority of the blood from the CCA to the brain. Because the function of the ICA is to supply the anterior and middle regions of the brain with oxygenated blood, it does so by its two terminal segments known as the anterior cerebral and middle cerebral arteries. The typical spectral waveform of a normal ICA will demonstrate a low-resistance, monophasic waveform when evaluated with

Copyright © Mometrix Media. You have been licensed one copy of this document for personal use only. Any other reproduction or redistribution is strictly prohibited. All rights reserved.
This content is provided for test preparation purposes only and does not imply an endorsement by Mometrix of any particular political, scientific, or religious point of view.

spectral Doppler. Blood flow within the ICA should also be noted as continuous flow through diastole.

Discerning Between the ICA or ECA

When performing a carotid duplex exam, there are several elements that may help the vascular technologist discern between the ICA and ECA. It is important to understand the location of these vessels and to consider what organs or tissues they supply. For example, the ECA supplies oxygenated blood to the face, scalp, and neck and tends to be situated more medially than the ICA. The ICA provides blood flow to the brain and is found in a more lateral position of the neck. The ECA has several extracranial branches that can be seen during the exam in comparison to the ICA, which only has intracranial branches. Along with the branches, the ECA is typically smaller compared to the ICA. However, the most dependable method is to use spectral Doppler. The ECA will demonstrate a rapid upstroke and downstroke during systole, less flow in diastole, and high-resistance blood flow in comparison to the ICA, which will demonstrate a waveform that is of low resistance.

Spectral Waveform When Performing a Carotid Duplex Study

The CCA supplies oxygenated blood to the head and neck regions. Most of the blood that travels through the CCA is directed into the ICA, which continuously feeds the brain with oxygenated blood. The continual supply of blood must occur amid the entire cardiac cycle, so a normal CCA should have a tracing that displays a moderately broad systolic peak as well as a moderate amount of diastolic flow. However, the blood that does not enter the ICA moves into the ECA, so the CCA has characteristics of both vessels that results in low- and high-resistance flow.

Blood Flow in the Posterolateral Portion of the Carotid Bulb

The carotid bulb is found in the distal portion of the CCA before the artery bifurcates into the ICA and the ECA. The carotid bulb is also referred to as the carotid sinus and is an area in which a noticeable dilation of the blood vessel may be visualized in the region of or just prior to the carotid bifurcation. When arteries are straight, the blood flow tends to display laminar flow. However, even without the presence of disease, the natural curve of the carotid bulb can cause a disturbance of flow in which separation occurs. The diameter of the carotid bulb as well as the divergence of the ICA and ECA origins can attribute to more pronounced flow separations.

Flow Characteristics of a Vertebral Artery That Is Unremarkable

The paired vertebral arteries ascend from the subclavian arteries on both sides of the neck to pass through the foramen magnum to eventually join to form the basilar artery. The basilar artery helps to supply the posterior region of the brain with oxygenated blood. The brain must have blood delivered to it continuously, so the flow patterns in the vertebral arteries should demonstrate low-resistance flow with continuous flow during diastole similar to that seen in the ICA because it also supplies the brain. The Doppler tracing should demonstrate flow that is moving toward the brain (antegrade).

Copyright © Mometrix Media. You have been licensed one copy of this document for personal use only. Any other reproduction or redistribution is strictly prohibited. All rights reserved.
This content is provided for test preparation purposes only and does not imply an endorsement by Mometrix of any particular political, scientific, or religious point of view.

Intracranial Cerebrovascular Exams

Brain's Anterior Circulation vs. Posterior Circulation

The brain requires a constant supply of oxygenated blood in order to function, which demands blood from two sources. These two sources are intracranial in location but receive their blood from extracranial blood vessels. The anterior system supplies blood to the ophthalmic artery as well as the cerebrum from the ICAs. The anterior cerebral arteries (ACAs) and middle cerebral arteries (MCAs) arise from the ICA and create a vascular channel that has low resistance because of the constant supply of blood that is required. These vessels help establish the circle of Willis. The posterior circulatory system supplies the occipital lobe, cerebellum, and brain stem, which are all located in the posterior region of the cranium. Recall that the bilateral vertebral arteries join to form the basilar artery (known as the vertebrobasilar system), which gives rise to the posterior cerebral arteries (PCAs) to help establish the circle of Willis.

Middle Cerebral Artery

The ICA enters the cranium on the right and left sides where it eventually bifurcates into the anterior cerebral arteries (ACAs) as well as the middle cerebral arteries (MCAs) at the terminal intracranial portion of the ICA. The MCA follows a more lateral projection in order to feed the cerebral cortex on the lateral sides of the brain. The MCA is often greater in diameter when compared to the ACA, and it is part of the anterior cerebrovascular circulatory system that supplies the brain with oxygenated blood. It is important for vascular technologists to realize that a large percentage of cerebrovascular accidents (CVAs) occur because the MCA has a high occlusion rate.

Circle of Willis

At the base of the brain, there is a network of vessels that is an anastomosis between the anterior and posterior circulatory systems of the brain. This channel connects the distal internal carotid, anterior, and posterior cerebral arteries via the anterior and posterior communicating arteries. The size of the circle of Willis is slightly larger than a quarter, and it resembles the shape of a hexagon. The circle of Willis is prone to congenital anomalies such as the development of a partial network in roughly 50% of patients, and many of the vessels are not symmetrical in size when compared to the contralateral side. In patients who do have a complete channel, it can serve as a collateral conduit in case one of the arteries on either the right or left side becomes blocked. The anterior and posterior communicating arteries serve as important collaterals if the extracranial arterial segments demonstrate significant stenosis.

Evaluation of the ACA with TCD

The anterior cerebral artery (ACA) begins when the distal ICA bifurcates within the cranium. These vessels are found bilaterally and are part of the anterior cerebrovascular system that supplies oxygenated blood to the brain and forms part of the circle of Willis. When assessing the ACA with transcranial Doppler (TCD), it is important to find the best window to insonate the vessel of interest. The

Copyright © Mometrix Media. You have been licensed one copy of this document for personal use only. Any other reproduction or redistribution is strictly prohibited. All rights reserved.
This content is provided for test preparation purposes only and does not imply an endorsement by Mometrix of any particular political, scientific, or religious point of view.

transtemporal window may be used to evaluate the flow within the ACA, and from this level, normal flow should be away from the transducer because it is moving to the front of the patient's brain. The mean velocity of blood flow in the ACA is 50 ± 11 cm/s.

Blood Flow in a Normal MCA Using TCD

The bifurcation of the intracranial portion of the distal ICA gives way to two vessels: the MCA and the ACA. The MCA is the bigger of the two divisions that is part of the anterior cerebrovascular system. The MCA supplies blood to the lateral portions of the brain. Due to the location of the MCA, the best window during a TCD will be the transtemporal window. The transducer is placed on the side of the patient's head, and the first tracing encountered is usually the MCA. The direction of blood flow at this point should be toward the transducer. The velocity of a normal MCA will be 55 ± 12 cm/s.

Window Used to Insonate the PCA Using TCD

The posterior cerebral arteries (PCAs) are bilateral vessels that are formed from the bifurcation of the basilar artery to supply the occipital lobe and a portion of the temporal lobes of the brain with oxygenated blood. The PCAs help complete the circle of Willis and can be evaluated via the temporal window with TCD. To find the PCA, it may be helpful to find where the distal ICA splits into the middle and ACAs and angle the transducer posteriorly and inferiorly. Because the PCA curves, the waveform will first be directed toward the probe and then course away from the transducer in the second part of the vessel. The velocity of the PCA is normally 40 ± 10 cm/s.

Depths and Velocities of Vessels

Terminal internal carotid artery (tICA), anterior cerebral artery (ACA), middle cerebral artery (MCA), posterior cerebral artery (PCA):

Artery	Direction of blood flow in comparison to the transducer	Depth	Normal velocity
tICA	Toward and/or away	60–70 mm	39 ± 9 cm/s
ACA	Away	60–75 mm	50 ± 11 cm/s
MCA	First segment toward; second segment away	30–60 mm	55 ± 12 cm/s
PCA	First segment toward; second segment away	60–75 mm	40 ± 10 cm/s

Window Used During TCD to Visualize the Vertebral Arteries

Recall that the vertebral arteries are situated in a more posterior location as they move superiorly from the clavicles toward the brain, passing through the cervical transverse foramen. To access the posterior region, it is helpful to use the suboccipital window. This can be obtained by having the patient roll onto his or her

Copyright © Mometrix Media. You have been licensed one copy of this document for personal use only. Any other reproduction or redistribution is strictly prohibited. All rights reserved.
This content is provided for test preparation purposes only and does not imply an endorsement by Mometrix of any particular political, scientific, or religious point of view.

side facing away from the sonographer and asking the patient to tuck their chin toward the chest. The transducer can be placed on the middle of the posterior neck just below the skull. The sonographer can then angle the beam up through the foramen magnum to better visualize the vertebral arteries. The vertebral arteries take on the appearance of a V shape before they unite to become the basilar artery. Flow in the vertebral arteries should move in a direction away from the transducer. The basilar artery can also be examined via the suboccipital window.

VEIN MAPPING

Vein mapping is performed when the patient is scheduled for a coronary artery bypass graft or if a dialysis site is needed. Deep veins are not harvested as bypass vessels, so only those in the superficial system are examined. The great saphenous vein (GSV), which is the longest vein in the body, is often the first vessel to be interrogated; it is found in the medial portion of the leg and courses from the top of the foot to the groin. If the GSV is not suitable for a bypass graft, then the small saphenous vein (SSV) may be used instead. However, if neither saphenous vein can be used due to disease within, small size, or if it has already been removed, the vascular technologist should evaluate the superficial veins of the upper extremities. The cephalic vein, which is found in the lateral portion of the upper extremity, is the preferred vessel, but the basilic vein could also be used.

Copyright © Mometrix Media. You have been licensed one copy of this document for personal use only. Any other reproduction or redistribution is strictly prohibited. All rights reserved.
This content is provided for test preparation purposes only and does not imply an endorsement by Mometrix of any particular political, scientific, or religious point of view.

Pathology, Perfusion, and Function

Aortoiliac Disease

Complications Experienced by a Patient with a Known AAA

The aorta is the blood vessel that transports oxygenated blood from the left ventricle of the heart to all cells in the body. After the aorta passes through the diaphragm, it becomes the abdominal aorta, which bifurcates at the level of the fourth lumbar vertebra. Abdominal aortic aneurysms (AAAs) are frequently diagnosed sonographically, with nearly 30% being diagnosed as an incidental finding. Aneurysm rupture is a major complication. The probability of rupture increases when a patient is a smoker. Other complications include distal embolization, especially aneurysms seen in the extremities, but this could stem from the abdominal aorta as well. Individuals with an aneurysm are more prone to developing another aneurysm often in the popliteal or common femoral arteries. If a vascular technologist diagnoses a unilateral popliteal artery aneurysm, it may be beneficial to evaluate the contralateral popliteal artery because bilateral presence is not uncommon.

Size of the Aneurysm Warranting Surgical Repair

The aorta is the largest artery in the human body. After the aorta descends through the diaphragm, it becomes the abdominal aorta. The average diameter of the abdominal aorta in adults is approximately 2 cm narrowing slightly as it descends toward the aortic bifurcation. Women tend to have an aorta that is somewhat smaller than men, usually measuring 2–3 mm less. This is important to consider because an aorta that measures more than 3 cm is considered an AAA. Another characterization of an AAA is when the region is 1.5 times the diameter of the segment that is just proximal in location. If the AAA has a measurement of 5.5 cm, then surgical repair is warranted because those that are larger than 6 cm have a 10%–20% risk of rupture. A 20%–40% chance of rupture accompanies an AAA that is 7 cm.

Fusiform vs. Saccular Aneurysms

An aneurysm is a dilation of an artery due to a weakness in the arterial wall that may develop in any artery. Abdominal aortic aneurysms, otherwise referred to as AAAs, materialize in the abdominal aorta and are diagnosed when the aorta measures more than 3 cm from outer wall to outer wall. Aneurysms are described to be fusiform when a focal segment of the blood vessel expands or bulges on all sides. Fusiform aneurysms tend to be the most common shape identified in aortic aneurysms, and they have ends that appear tapered. Another shape created by an aortic aneurysm is called a saccular aneurysm. This type often occurs when the patient has experienced trauma. The dilation is asymmetrical because it only occurs on one side of the vessel and tends to transpire in the thoracic aorta more often than the abdominal portion.

Copyright © Mometrix Media. You have been licensed one copy of this document for personal use only. Any other reproduction or redistribution is strictly prohibited. All rights reserved.
This content is provided for test preparation purposes only and does not imply an endorsement by Mometrix of any particular political, scientific, or religious point of view.

Measuring an Aneurysm

Ultrasound is the imaging modality of choice when performing abdominal aortic screenings for AAAs or as a follow-up method when an AAA was previously diagnosed with ultrasound or any other modality such as CT, MRI, or X-ray. An aneurysm is diagnosed when either a dilation of the artery is more than 3 cm or if a bulge seen has a diameter of 1.5 times more than a connecting segment of the aorta. Longitudinal and transverse images with AP measurements should be taken in the proximal, mid, and distal regions of the abdominal aorta. When an AAA is discovered during an ultrasound exam, the technologist should carefully document the location and size by measuring the aneurysm from outer wall to outer wall. In the transverse plane, the maximum diameter should be documented. It is not important to measure the length of the aneurysm, but it should be documented if the iliac arteries are also affected.

Aortic Dissection

An aortic dissection is a life-threatening condition that develops when there is a tear in the innermost layer of the arterial wall (referred to as the intima). This tear enables blood to seep into a false lumen, which is created between the inner and middle layers of the artery. When the true and false lumens are evaluated with color and spectral Doppler, they could demonstrate different directions and velocities. The false lumen will often demonstrate bidirectional, high-resistance flow, whereas normal spectral waveforms may be seen in the true lumen. Ultrasound findings will also display a hyperechoic flap or membrane that separates the true and false lumens. If the false lumen clots, no blood flow would be demonstrated with color Doppler. The thoracic aorta is the region in which dissections typically develop, but they can continue into the abdominal and even the iliac arteries. People that have Marfan syndrome are genetically predisposed to aortic dissections as are those that experience trauma.

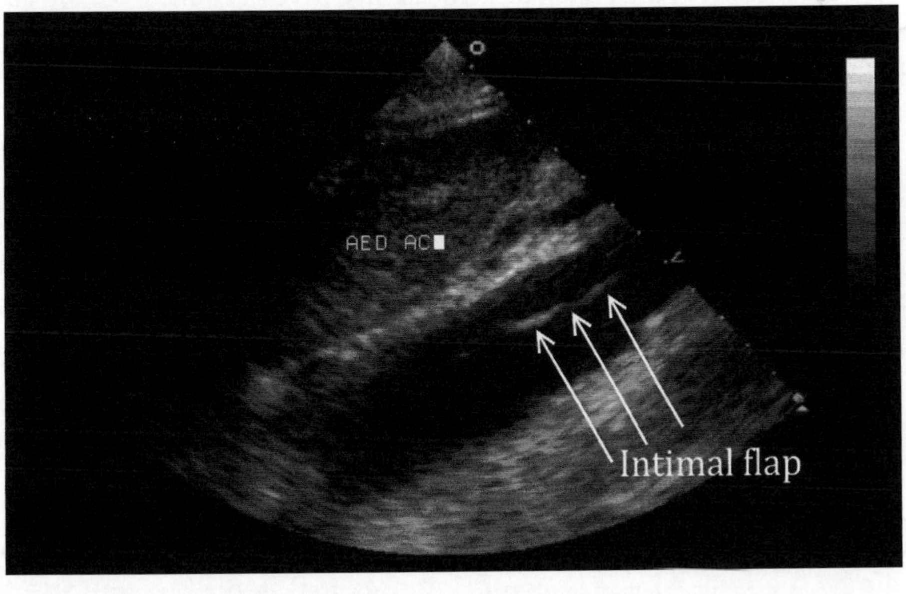

Copyright © Mometrix Media. You have been licensed one copy of this document for personal use only. Any other reproduction or redistribution is strictly prohibited. All rights reserved.
This content is provided for test preparation purposes only and does not imply an endorsement by Mometrix of any particular political, scientific, or religious point of view.

Aortic Ectasia

Ectasia of the aorta is suspected when there is a general dilation of the artery that has not yet reached aneurysmal dimensions. A standard measurement of the abdominal aorta is 3 cm or less when measured from outer wall to outer wall or if the diameter is 1.5 times less than what the more proximal connecting segment of the abdominal aorta measures. Individuals that have been diagnosed with ectasia have a higher incidence of developing an aneurysm because this swelling may continue to evolve; follow-up ultrasounds are often performed to evaluate this progression. Ectasia of the aorta may be seen when interrogating the thoracic, abdominal, and even the common iliac arteries.

Using Extended Field of View Control

When the vascular technologist would like to visualize as much of the abdominal aorta as possible at one time, the extended field of view control on the ultrasound system should be used. This panoramic image is available on most modern ultrasound equipment, and it replaces the split-screen method of demonstrating objects that are longer than the transducer face. By acquiring various volume data, the system will stitch the information together in order to display one image. This single image will offer clinicians the ability to visualize the majority of the structure at the same time. This application can be used when interrogating the abdominal aorta, and it may provide additional information regarding the exact location of aneurysms or ectasia that may be encountered. Often, anatomical structures are enlarged and may be difficult to obtain measurements from.

Signal Found in the CFA If Significant Aortoiliac Lesion

It is essential to correctly diagnose patients that have aortoiliac lesions to aid in the treatment of peripheral arterial disease (PAD). In some cases, the distal region of the aorta and the proximal portion of the common iliac arteries are difficult to evaluate well due to bowel gas and the depth of these structures. Evaluation of the common femoral artery (CFA) may be useful when Doppler evaluation of the aortoiliac region is not possible. Spectral Doppler of a normal CFA will demonstrate a waveform that is triphasic with a reversal of flow seen below the baseline with a clean spectral window. In patients that present with a significant aortoiliac lesion, the CFA waveform will appear monophasic. If there is a total proximal occlusion, then collaterals feed the extremities and demonstrate a dampened signal as long as the occlusion was not acute.

Waveform That Demonstrates Tardus Parvus

Tardus parvus is a term that is used to describe how a pulse-wave spectral Doppler waveform appears when there is a more proximal stenosis present. Characteristics of a tardus parvus waveform include a delayed acceleration (which is also often referred to as a slow upstroke). The waveform will also have a more rounded (dampened) peak systolic appearance. This pattern could be seen in the left common iliac artery if there is an obstruction of the abdominal aorta. This pattern is also commonly seen when there is significant proximal stenosis of any artery in the

Copyright © Mometrix Media. You have been licensed one copy of this document for personal use only. Any other reproduction or redistribution is strictly prohibited. All rights reserved.
This content is provided for test preparation purposes only and does not imply an endorsement by Mometrix of any particular political, scientific, or religious point of view.

body. Tardus parvus is commonly seen distal to a stenosis in the renal artery or if collateral channels have formed in the case of a total arterial occlusion.

Region of Abdominal Aorta with the Highest Incidence of Aneurysms

When a vascular technologist is evaluating the abdominal aorta, longitudinal and transverse images with measurements should be performed. Proximal images and measurements should be taken in the vicinity of the origin of the celiac artery below the diaphragm. The region in which the renal arteries start is where the measurements should be labeled as mid aorta. The distal region of the abdominal aorta is measured just prior to where the aorta bifurcates to become the right and left common iliac arteries. The majority of AAAs are found in the distal segment of the abdominal aorta and considered to be infrarenal in location. Infrarenal describes the area below the origin of the renal arteries.

Pseudoaneurysm

A pseudoaneurysm can result from any endovascular procedure, angiography, or the use of a dialysis access site. These are formed when blood seeps out of the artery and into the neighboring tissues. Patients may complain of a pulsatile, painful mass that appears red. The neck of this "false aneurysm" is the pathway that allows the blood to escape from the artery into the main capsule. Although some of these will resolve on their own, others will require procedures to create a clot. Some options for treatment include ultrasound-guided manual compression and injections. When injections are used, thrombin is instilled into the pocket to create a hematoma. Surgical repair is warranted when the artery is greatly damaged.

Coarctation of the Aorta

Coarctation of the aorta is a congenital heart defect that develops because of a constriction of or the narrowing of the aorta. This narrowing often develops distal to the origin point of the left subclavian artery and may be found in conjunction with other heart conditions, but it can also affect the abdominal aorta. Depending on the severity of this narrowing of the aorta, the patient may be diagnosed at different ages and a mild case may not be diagnosed until the individual develops hypertension, whereas others are diagnosed with this condition shortly after birth. This narrowing can often be seen on gray-scale and color Doppler images. In children and young adults that have abnormal renal artery duplex studies in addition to high blood pressure, a coarctation of the aorta should be suspected.

Claudication

Claudication is pain in the extremities due to narrowing of the aorta or peripheral arteries, which is called peripheral arterial disease (PAD). Atherosclerosis is often the cause of claudication, which results in decreased blood flow to the extremities, especially during exercise. In the early stages, patients may describe their symptoms as pain or aching that often disappears during rest. As the narrowing of the vessels increases, patients may complain of pain even when resting. Other symptoms may include weakness of the limbs, skin discoloration and/or ulcers, or cold feet. The lower extremities are affected more often than the arms. The vessels that exhibit

Copyright © Mometrix Media. You have been licensed one copy of this document for personal use only. Any other reproduction or redistribution is strictly prohibited. All rights reserved.
This content is provided for test preparation purposes only and does not imply an endorsement by Mometrix of any particular political, scientific, or religious point of view.

atherosclerosis or arteriosclerosis are the femoral and popliteal arteries. Blockages can develop in the aorta and iliac vessels as well.

Claudication Location Symptoms

When patients experience claudication, the location of symptoms can often determine at which level the diseased arteries are located. For example, if the patient has pain on both sides of the buttocks, then it is assumed that there is significant disease of the distal aorta and or iliac arteries. If only one side is symptomatic, then unilateral iliofemoral disease is suspected of the ipsilateral (same) side.

Location of claudication symptoms	Type of disease present	Unilateral symptoms
Buttocks	Aortoiliac disease when pain is bilateral	The iliofemoral region is suspected when pain is unilateral.
Thigh	Distal external iliac/common femoral	This could be a unilateral finding.
Calf	Femoral/popliteal	This could be a unilateral finding.

Leriche Syndrome

Leriche syndrome is the result of an obstruction of the distal aorta that is typically found in males between the ages of 30 and 40. This is different from most cases of occlusive disease of the abdominal aorta because it is seen more often in older populations that have significant atherosclerosis. Acute and chronic cases have been diagnosed, with acute onset seen more often in females. Male patients with chronic cases of Leriche syndrome often present with the triad of decreased or absent femoral pulses; intermittent claudication of the pelvis, thighs, and calves; and erectile dysfunction. Still other symptoms include coldness of the lower extremities, pain, and numbness of the extremities. Over time, there is progression of the occlusion, which is typically proximal to the aortic bifurcation but may extend proximally and distally into the iliac and femoral arteries.

Venous Insufficiency

Oxygenated blood is carried away from the heart in arteries, whereas blood that has been depleted of oxygen is returned to the heart in blood vessels known as veins. Veins have internal structures known as valves that stem from the same tissue that makes up the innermost layer of the wall of the vein and assist in moving the blood toward the heart. These valves, when working correctly, also prevent blood flow from traveling in the wrong direction. Incompetent valves enable the blood to flow backward (as well as in a normal antegrade direction). This reflux precipitates pooling of blood in the legs, which leads to what is known as chronic venous insufficiency (CVI). Pressure within the vessels becomes increased, and fluid and blood may seep into the surrounding tissue, which is why people with CVI often

Copyright © Mometrix Media. You have been licensed one copy of this document for personal use only. Any other reproduction or redistribution is strictly prohibited. All rights reserved.
This content is provided for test preparation purposes only and does not imply an endorsement by Mometrix of any particular political, scientific, or religious point of view.

have a brown color in their limbs. Up to 75% of ulcers that develop in the lower extremity are due to CVI.

Importance of the Calf Muscle Pump

An important component of the lower extremities to preserve normal blood return to the heart is known as the calf muscle pump. This system is comprised of veins that serve as a storage receptacle for blood, calf muscles, and internal venous valves that are competent and able to ensure one-way blood flow. When a patient walks or flexes the foot, the muscles within the calf act as a pump that squeezes the veins as the muscles contract. The ejection fraction of this venous/skeletal pump should be greater than 60% to prevent venous insufficiency.

Veins, like arteries, have three separate layers that make up the wall of the blood vessels. The walls of veins are less muscular than those of arteries. The middle layer (adventitia media) of veins is the thinnest component. Because veins tend to be less muscular, they are less elastic than arteries. Veins dilate in patients with venous insufficiency due to the pooling of blood in the distal portions of the lower extremities. When blood starts to collect due to incompetent valves, venous stasis can occur and will also contribute to the dilation of calf veins. The rise of hydrostatic pressure can create an expansion of the veins as well.

Upper Extremity Venous Disease

Paget-Schroetter Syndrome

Thoracic outlet syndrome (TOS) may occur due to compression (or clotting) of veins, arteries, or nerves in the small area between the clavicle and first rib, which is known as the thoracic outlet. If this space tends to be more narrow than usual, compression of these structures and venous stasis can occur. Paget-Schroetter syndrome is part of the venous component of TOS and is typically created when the subclavian or axillary vein becomes clotted due to activities that involve the same or exaggerated motions of the upper extremities. Often, sports-related activities create repetitive movements that can stress these blood vessels and create a clot such as swimming, throwing a football or baseball, or lifting weights. Other non-sports-related injuries occur when people constantly lift or hold heavy items overhead or work on computers without giving their body the proper amount of time to rest. Paget-Schroetter syndrome is also referred to as stress or effort thrombosis; symptoms include pain in the shoulder or arm with or without numbness or tingling. People may also complain of weakness of the affected hand when trying to grab objects.

Flow Patterns When Examining the Subclavian Veins

The subclavian veins are found on each side of the body. The subclavian veins originate near the first rib once the axillary and cephalic veins merge. As the name implies, the subclavian vein travels underneath the clavicle and is anterior to the subclavian artery. The subclavian vein tends to demonstrate pulsatile venous flow due to a location that is in close proximity to the heart. Along with cardiac pulsations, veins that are situated closer to the heart also demonstrate respiratory

Copyright © Mometrix Media. You have been licensed one copy of this document for personal use only. Any other reproduction or redistribution is strictly prohibited. All rights reserved.
This content is provided for test preparation purposes only and does not imply an endorsement by Mometrix of any particular political, scientific, or religious point of view.

patterns. The internal jugular, brachiocephalic, and subclavian veins all have similar waveforms. As the vessels travel further away from the heart such as those found in the lower extremities, the vessels are compressible (as long as there is not a blood clot) and have spontaneous, phasic flow. When the distal extremity is squeezed, augmentation will be exhibited.

No Demonstration of Pulsatile Flow

Vascular technologists should expect to see pulsatile flow when evaluating the subclavian vein with spectral Doppler. This pulsatility occurs because the subclavian vein is positioned close to the heart. If the subclavian vein does not demonstrate phasic, pulsatile flow, then it is assumed that there is an obstruction proximal to the subclavian vein on the side being evaluated. Often, the flow in this case will become continuous in addition to the loss of pulsatility. Due to the bony anatomy around the subclavian and brachiocephalic veins, it can be difficult to perform compression when ruling out a DVT, so it is important to use color and spectral Doppler for evaluation, which is why it is important to understand the normal waveforms of veins that are close to the heart. Always evaluate for the presence of echogenic material within the lumen of the blood vessel as well as collaterals that may have developed.

Lower Extremity Venous Disease

Common Ultrasound Characteristics of a DVT

The common ultrasound appearance of a deep vein thrombosis (DVT) is a vein that is dilated. During a venous duplex ultrasound, the vascular technologist will not be able to compress the vein wall to wall. The vascular technologist may notice during the exam that the thrombus does not appear to be completely attached to the wall of the blood vessel (this may be more noticeable in the sagittal plane when scanning the distal portion of the thrombus because motion may be discerned). An acute DVT may appear more hypoechoic than a chronic clot, which tends to be more echogenic. Often with chronic changes, synechiae will be apparent within the affected vessel(s), which represent the lysis and contraction of the clot. The arrow in this ultrasound

Copyright © Mometrix Media. You have been licensed one copy of this document for personal use only. Any other reproduction or redistribution is strictly prohibited. All rights reserved.
This content is provided for test preparation purposes only and does not imply an endorsement by Mometrix of any particular political, scientific, or religious point of view.

image demonstrates a thrombus that is present in the left CFV. Chronic clots may also demonstrate recanalized and/or collateral vessels.

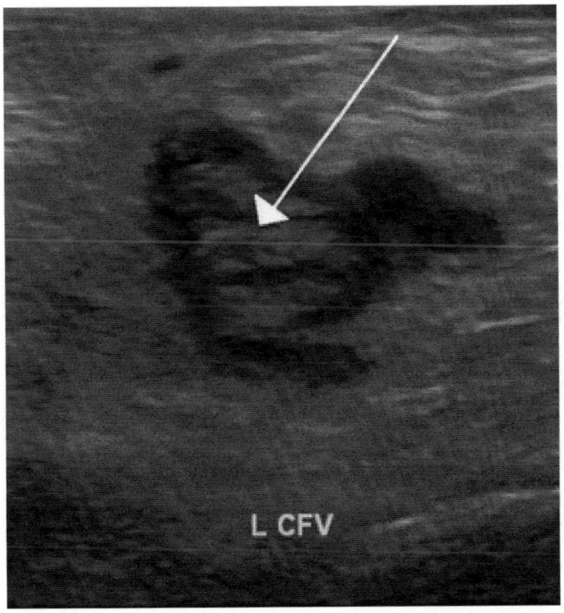

https://upload.wikimedia.org/wikipedia/commons/thumb/b/bd/dvtus.png/284px-dvtus.png

Main Clinical Concern with a DVT

If a patient develops an acute DVT, the main clinical concern is a pulmonary embolism (PE). A PE occurs when part of the thrombus, or in some cases the entire clot, breaks off and travels within the circulatory system and becomes lodged in one of the pulmonary arteries, which can be fatal. In cases that are not fatal, damage to the lungs or other organs can occur because the amount of oxygenated blood is reduced due to the obstruction. Patients that have a PE will often present with shortness of breath or chest pain. Typically, a PE is the result of a DVT in the lower extremities. The symptoms of a DVT in the extremities often include pain, swelling, warmth, and redness. DVTs can occur when an individual does not move for long periods of time such as after long flights or even after surgery. Some patients develop them because of hormone-related medicines such as birth control. Other individuals have a genetic predisposition to blood clots.

CVI Common for Those with a Previous DVT

In patients that have had a previous DVT, the most common complication is chronic venous insufficiency ([CVI] a pulmonary embolism is the most severe life-threatening complication). This is also referred to as post-thrombotic syndrome when venous insufficiency occurs because of a blood clot. If a DVT forms and propagates, it can cause permanent distension of the walls of the veins while creating scar tissue within the blood vessel itself. This scar tissue can extend to the internal valves, which creates the inability to ensure one-way blood flow (valvular incompetence). When the direction of blood flow within the veins no longer only propagates toward the heart, the blood can pool within the vessels, which increases

Copyright © Mometrix Media. You have been licensed one copy of this document for personal use only. Any other reproduction or redistribution is strictly prohibited. All rights reserved.
This content is provided for test preparation purposes only and does not imply an endorsement by Mometrix of any particular political, scientific, or religious point of view.

the amount of venous pressure. The calf and ankle area often become edematous because of blood, fluids, and fibrinogen escaping into the adjacent tissues because of the rise in venous pressure.

Source of Thrombosis When a Patient Experiences a PE

A PE typically derives from a DVT of the lower extremities. Although not all clinicians agree about the treatment and management of DVTs when found in the lower leg, the most common source of thrombosis, which causes deadly PE, is the soleal vein. This occurrence takes place because the soleal muscle only functions in the area of the ankle (unlike the gastrocnemius muscle, which functions throughout the entire lower leg). When individuals are not able to move either because of an injury or an inability to walk, or if they are on a long car ride or flight, the soleal vein can become sluggish and not drain normally because it is not contracting. The soleal veins drain into the peroneal and posterior tibial veins.

Soleal and Gastrocnemius Veins

The calf muscles have two groups of veins that return blood to the heart, which have the same name as the muscles that make up the calf (soleal and gastrocnemius veins). It is important to note that these veins drain into separate deep vessels. The soleal vein returns blood into the peroneal and posterior tibial veins via 10 or more sinusoids. The two segments of the gastrocnemius vein exit both heads of the gastrocnemius muscles and empty into the medial and lateral portions of popliteal vein. If a patient develops a DVT within the gastrocnemius vein, it is important during a venous duplex follow-up exam to determine if the blood clot has propagated into the popliteal vein, which is one of the larger deep veins. If the blood clot is only within one of the calf muscle veins, it is referred to as an isolated calf muscle thrombosis.

Development of Venous Ulcers

Ulcers are open wounds or sores that develop when there is an interruption of circulation to parts of the body. Ulcers may be the result of venous and/or arterial disease such as CVI or PAD. Venous ulcers materialize when there is valvular incompetency and the blood pools in the lower leg and ankle area. Edema and venous hypertension are responsible for the typical location of these venous ulcers because they are found most of the time in the region known as the gaiter zone, which is the area just above the medial and lateral malleoli. In the area of the medial malleolus, several important perforators are found, which is why the tissue breakdown is evident here. Ulcers of venous origin in this area do not typically hurt as much as those that stem from arterial disease. However, these ulcers do tend to ooze, and if the ulcers are characterized as "wet," they are associated as venous stasis ulcers, which have a high correlation with venous insufficiency.

Comparing the Phasicity of Both Sides

A vascular technologist should perform a complete venous duplex exam on the affected side to rule out a DVT for swelling, even if the exam is negative for a DVT from the CFV distally. However, the protocol for a unilateral exam should include a

Copyright © Mometrix Media. You have been licensed one copy of this document for personal use only. Any other reproduction or redistribution is strictly prohibited. All rights reserved.
This content is provided for test preparation purposes only and does not imply an endorsement by Mometrix of any particular political, scientific, or religious point of view.

spectral Doppler waveform of the contralateral side (CFV) to compare phasicity signals. The vascular technologist should perform this comparison while scanning in the long axis with the patient in the exact same position that the affected side was scanned. If there is a discrepancy noted with phasicity or if the waveform appears continuous, which means it isn't affected at all during respiration, then it is important to look for an obstruction in a more proximal location. Some labs may require both external iliac veins to also be interrogated to compare respiratory phasicity. If a patient has an obstructive thrombosis of the iliofemoral veins, it can cause pallor and excessive swelling; this is a condition referred to as phlegmasia alba dolens.

Managing CVI

It is important to diagnose and manage CVI as quickly as possible before tissues break down and ulcers develop. Patients need to understand the importance of proper nutrition, exercise, and taking steps to care for their skin. When skin infections are present, antibiotics may need to be prescribed. Individuals with CVI must avoid sitting for extended periods to prevent the blood from pooling in the lower legs. Also, the patient should try to rest with their feet up after it is necessary to be on their feet. Physicians may prescribe compression stockings as well. If ulcers are already present, medicated (Unna) boots and dressings may be the first treatment step. If these are not effective, the patient may need to be treated with several sessions of hyperbaric oxygen therapy.

Primary and Secondary Varicose Veins

Varicose veins appear as tortuous, enlarged veins that develop when these vessels become overdistended with blood and allow pooling within. Veins that work normally tend to allow the propagation of blood flow from the lower extremities to the heart. When valves no longer work properly, retrograde flow tends to cause enlargement of the veins. Primary varicose veins are diagnosed when only the superficial system is affected by valvular incompetence. Sometimes, this is due to the congenital absence of valves, which can cause an increase of the venous pressure that does not affect the deep veins. Secondary varicose veins, however, do involve the deep venous system. These circumstances could include a prior DVT, which in turn damages the valves to allow retrograde flow. Secondary varicose veins also involve the incompetence of the superficial valves as well.

Scenario

Spectral Doppler demonstrates continuous flow of the popliteal vein in a patient that presents with pain in the calf and associated swelling. The patient also describes a fullness in the popliteal fossa. Explain if this would likely be a positive or negative venous duplex study and what else the vascular technologist should evaluate for.

In a patient that presents with a fullness in the popliteal fossa and continuous flow of the popliteal vein when examined with spectral Doppler, the vascular technologist should also evaluate the popliteal fossa. The fullness behind the knee, pain, and swelling could be caused by a Baker's cyst. A Baker's cyst can create a fluid

Copyright © Mometrix Media. You have been licensed one copy of this document for personal use only. Any other reproduction or redistribution is strictly prohibited. All rights reserved.
This content is provided for test preparation purposes only and does not imply an endorsement by Mometrix of any particular political, scientific, or religious point of view.

collection in the posteromedial portion of the knee joint, which could compress the popliteal vein to cause the continuous signal within. If a dedicated venous duplex exam was also performed, it would likely be negative for DVT because a ruptured Baker's cyst can cause pain and swelling of the calf.

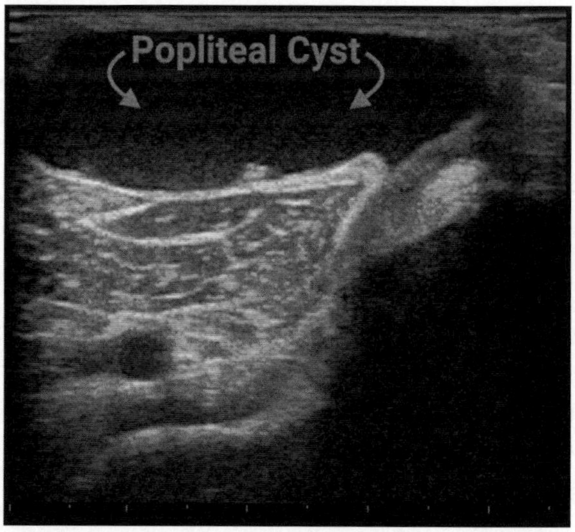

Improving Color Doppler Images with Persistence

Persistence is an averaging technique that will combine images from older frames with those of newer data. In gray-scale imaging, persistence can be used to smooth out an image or reduce the amount of noise that is present. Persistence is also found to be useful in color Doppler imaging, especially if the vessels to be visualized are deeper in the body (such as in cases of obese patients or edema), to identify vessels that contain slow-moving blood, or if there is an obstruction of a vessel. Smaller blood vessels can also be identified more readily than with methods that do not implement persistence. It is important to note that the temporal resolution is often decreased when persistence is applied to an image.

Ascending vs. Descending Venography Exams

Venograms require the use of contrast to be injected and X-ray equipment to take sequential images of the veins. These exams can be uncomfortable for patients and require extreme technical expertise to read and perform the exams. Ascending venography can be used in the upper and lower extremities, whereas descending venography is only performed of the lower extremities. During an ascending venogram, the physician will inject the contrast into either the basilic or cephalic vein for the upper extremities and into a vein on the top of the foot if the lower extremity is being examined. Ascending venography can determine if a DVT or varicosities are present, if the patient has had previous blood clots, and the presence of collateral vessels. A descending venogram requires injection of contrast via the common femoral vein to assess the function of the valves (venous incompetence) as well as assessing for reflux.

Copyright © Mometrix Media. You have been licensed one copy of this document for personal use only. Any other reproduction or redistribution is strictly prohibited. All rights reserved.
This content is provided for test preparation purposes only and does not imply an endorsement by Mometrix of any particular political, scientific, or religious point of view.

NATIVE UPPER EXTREMITY ARTERY DISEASE

SIGNS TO AID IN THE DIAGNOSIS OF TOS

Thoracic outlet syndrome (TOS) may occur due to factors related to arterial or venous complications. Although roughly 30% of people with TOS do not experience any symptoms, others present with pain in the shoulder or upper arm further accompanied by numbness and/or tingling. Other individuals may notice a decrease in the force of their grip. Patients may notice that this pain or numbness intensifies when working out, especially when their arm is in certain raised positions. Vascular technologists should prove that flow is at least reduced (because it is not always absent) when scanning the patient in different positions. Notably, the patient may be suffering from disorders related to the cervical spine or carpal tunnel because they may provoke similar symptoms.

BUERGER'S DISEASE

Buerger's disease, also referred to as thrombosis obliterans, is the most common type of arteritis. Arteritis occurs when the walls of the artery become inflamed, which can create a distal occlusion of the arteries within the fingers and toes due to a blood clot. Buerger's disease is almost always found in younger men between the ages of 20 and 40 that are heavy smokers or use chewing tobacco. It is assumed that the chemicals in cigarettes and chewing tobacco create swelling of the blood vessels. Claudication is a common symptom that patients experience as well as numbness and/or tingling of the fingers or toes. The fingers or toes may have ulcers or gangrene, which can lead to their amputation.

RAYNAUD'S PHENOMENON

Raynaud's phenomenon can affect the fingers or toes when the blood supply to these regions is obstructed. There are two types of Raynaud's phenomenon, with the first being known as primary or idiopathic, which occurs intermittently in generally healthy patients. This stems from vasospasms within the hand and feet that supply oxygenated blood to the digits. This form is believed to be hereditary and is common in young women especially when exposed to cold temperatures. Primary Raynaud's usually presents as discoloration of the digits bilaterally but with little to no pain. The prognosis tends to be positive for these individuals. Secondary Raynaud's is also known as obstructive Raynaud's and is the result of other underlying medical conditions such as autoimmune diseases or arthritis. Unlike the primary form of this disease, the ischemia always exists, and patients may have excruciating pain, numbness, and tingling due to an arterial obstruction that is constant even though the arterioles constrict normally.

NATIVE LOWER EXTREMITY ARTERY DISEASE

PREVAILING VESSEL IN WHICH ATHEROSCLEROSIS DEVELOPS

In healthy patients, arteries demonstrate elasticity to move the blood throughout the circulatory system with the contractions of the heart. Arteriosclerosis takes place when the arterial walls no longer have the same elasticity. Atherosclerosis can be defined as plaque accumulation within the arteries due to damage to the arterial wall. This plaque can be comprised of cholesterol or fats and can restrict the flow of

Copyright © Mometrix Media. You have been licensed one copy of this document for personal use only. Any other reproduction or redistribution is strictly prohibited. All rights reserved.
This content is provided for test preparation purposes only and does not imply an endorsement by Mometrix of any particular political, scientific, or religious point of view.

oxygen-rich blood to vital organs. Risk factors of arterial disease include smoking, hypertension, diabetes, high cholesterol, and high triglycerides. These plaques can also break off or erupt, initiating a DVT. Atherosclerosis can develop in any artery, but this condition typically occurs in the brachiocephalic vessel, carotid bifurcation, infrarenal aorta, and iliac and femoral arteries. Atherosclerosis is visualized in the distal femoral artery more often than in other arteries.

Appearance of Adequate Blood Flow Volume at Rest

When a patient is resting, there are various reasons why the volume of blood flow seems adequate even when there is a hemodynamically significant stenosis present. The first reason is that when a patient is resting, the amount of peripheral resistance will be less than that if the patient is active. Vasodilation, or a widening of the arteries, will allow more blood to pass through a vessel. However, if a person is exercising, the elevation of the pulse will create arterial constriction so the blood feeds the muscles with oxygenated blood. Another reason for an apparent normal volume of flow when the patient has a hemodynamically significant stenosis is the formation of collateral channels, which enables the blood to flow around the part of the artery that is stenosed.

Blue Toe Syndrome

If a patient presents to the emergency department or physician's office with a blue toe(s), the provider should consider blue toe syndrome. This condition will cause the toes to have a cyanotic appearance. This bluish/purplish discoloration is caused when small blood vessels are blocked by some sort of emboli. Mechanical obstruction can be caused when a thrombus breaks off, and the emboli become lodged in the tiny distal arteries of the toes. These emboli are primarily the result of atherosclerosis and are the main concern when a peripheral aneurysm is present in one of the arteries. These emboli could also be caused from gases or liquids such as contrast that was injected during an angiographic exam or anticoagulant treatment. Collateral arterial channels may form, which will alleviate the ischemia and discoloration of the affected digits.

Popliteal Entrapment Syndrome

Popliteal entrapment syndrome is caused when the popliteal artery is compressed by the head of the gastrocnemius muscle, which, when contracted, decreases blood flow to the lower portion of the leg. This condition may be the result of a congenital anomaly of the gastrocnemius muscle, or it may develop as a result of athletic training and hypertrophy of the calf muscle (this can occur bilaterally). This condition typically arises in young men (often younger than the age of 30) who are athletes. If an active athlete describes symptoms of intermittent swelling, cramping, numbness, and aching during physical activity that disappear shortly after running, then the physician should consider popliteal entrapment syndrome even though this is a rare condition. When testing is performed, it should be done with and without muscle contraction for comparison, and if it is positive for entrapment a decrease of perfusion will be evident during contraction.

Copyright © Mometrix Media. You have been licensed one copy of this document for personal use only. Any other reproduction or redistribution is strictly prohibited. All rights reserved.
This content is provided for test preparation purposes only and does not imply an endorsement by Mometrix of any particular political, scientific, or religious point of view.

Arteriovenous Fistula

The circulatory system is a closed network of blood vessels that carries oxygenated blood to the cells of the body and returns blood that has been depleted of oxygen back to the heart. The blood travels through the body once it is pumped from the heart to the arteries, arterioles, capillaries, venules, and then to the veins. If blood passes directly from the arteries to the veins, it is known as an arteriovenous fistula (AVF). When the atypical assembly of these vessels occurs, it is important to diagnose this condition as quickly as possible because the regions that are fed by the capillaries receives a reduced blood supply preventing them from obtaining the proper amounts of nutrients and oxygen. Individuals that are undergoing dialysis may need to have a procedure in which an AVF is generated so that it can be used as an access site. AVFs may materialize on their own or as the result of trauma.

Arterial Ulcers

When an individual experiences a decrease in perfusion to the lower extremities, there is an increased risk of development of an arterial ulcer. An ulcer occurs when there is a breakdown of skin and tissue in any area of the body. This opening can increase the risk of infection because bacteria can easily enter the wound. Arterial ulcers typically occur as a result of atherosclerosis, which hinders the blood supply to the limb, which exacerbates the amount of damage to the surrounding region. Arterial ulcerations, when compared to venous ulcers, tend to cause a great deal of pain. Antibiotics are often necessary, and prompt diagnosis and management are necessary to increase circulation to that area. The location of arterial ulcers often involves the lower extremity, especially the toes and sometimes near the tibia. Although these wounds don't bleed very often, they are frequently very deep, and the skin may have a shiny appearance.

Determining the Location of Collateral Channels

Collateral channels develop in arteries so that blood can bypass the region that is totally occluded or shows significant stenosis to reach the more distal regions. It can be helpful to perform Doppler segmental pressures when complete occlusion of an artery is present to help identify the level at which the blockage has occurred. In cases of a significant stenosis or complete occlusion, collateral channels will often materialize, which will still allow for a normal amount of blood flow when the patient is resting. When a blockage has occurred, the blood flow patterns in collaterals that are near or at a more distant position could demonstrate increased velocities with a more pulsatile waveform and increased total volume of blood.

Associated Embolus with a Peripheral Arterial Aneurysm

When a lower extremity develops a peripheral arterial aneurysm, there is often an associated thrombus within the lumen aneurysm. This thrombus forms because the blood inside the dilated vessel tends to take on a back-and-forth whirling configuration. When part of the clot breaks off, it often travels distally and lodges within a smaller digital artery. An embolus (emboli) can interrupt the transportation of blood distally to the individual's limb because it may become obstructed, creating what is known as blue toe syndrome. Although a rupture of an

Copyright © Mometrix Media. You have been licensed one copy of this document for personal use only. Any other reproduction or redistribution is strictly prohibited. All rights reserved.
This content is provided for test preparation purposes only and does not imply an endorsement by Mometrix of any particular political, scientific, or religious point of view.

aneurysm of the abdominal aorta is the main concern, an embolism is the most common complication of a peripheral arterial aneurysm.

Effect of Hemodynamically Significant Stenosis

Laminar flow is the type of flow that is exhibited in patent blood vessels. If a clinician listens to the blood moving through a vessel with laminar flow, it will not be concerning. This flow is layered and smooth, and it travels parallel along the length of the vessel. If the diameter of the artery decreases by 50%, then it is assumed that the cross-sectional area has been decreased by 75% in the presence of a hemodynamically significant stenosis. When the diameter of the artery has been affected, the velocity of the blood flow will increase. If a provider hears an abnormal sound when listening with a stethoscope, this is known as a bruit. A bruit is caused by blood flow that is abnormally turbulent, but it may not be heard when a total occlusion or significant stenosis is present.

Spectral Broadening

A spectral Doppler waveform represents all of the velocities found in a sample of a blood within a particular vessel. Two types of flow can be ascertained in the sample. The first is normal, or laminar, flow, in which the spectral window is clear and the red blood cells are traveling at almost the same velocities. The second type of flow is turbulent flow, which shows movement that is disorganized because the blood is traveling at different speeds and various directions. Instead of a clear spectral window as seen in laminar flow, it appears to be filled in, which represents spectral broadening. Spectral broadening is a display of a broad range of Doppler shifts that are apparent within the sample of blood flow taken in a vessel. This may happen due to a stenotic or tortuous vessel.

Emergency of Acute Occlusion

If an acute occlusion is suspected of the lower extremities, it is considered an emergency because oxygenated blood is not reaching the entire lower extremity, which may cause a loss of function of the extremities. For example, if the patient's mid femoral artery is occluded, everything distal to that blood vessel (the distal thigh, knee, lower leg, and foot) won't receive the blood that it should, which can cause ischemia or tissue death. This is a very serious condition that requires immediate treatment such as bypass, thrombolysis, or even embolectomy. Chronic arterial disease is not considered an emergency, on the other hand, because the longer an artery is stenosed, there has likely been ample time for collateral channels to form. Collateral pathways enable blood to be rerouted to bypass the area of the artery that is affected by the occlusion so the distal extremity can still be supplied with oxygenated blood.

Ischemic Rest Pain

Severe toe pain is an indication of ischemic rest pain, which is closely affiliated with a severe form of PAD. The patient may also experience pain throughout their feet and even in the heels especially when they are in the resting position with their legs at or above the level of their heart. In this position, the patient may also notice their

Copyright © Mometrix Media. You have been licensed one copy of this document for personal use only. Any other reproduction or redistribution is strictly prohibited. All rights reserved.
This content is provided for test preparation purposes only and does not imply an endorsement by Mometrix of any particular political, scientific, or religious point of view.

feet changing from their normal color and becoming pale. Often, the pain dissipates when the individual sits or stands up, which allows blood flow to reach the feet once again. This change of positioning will also return the normal color to their feet as gravity enables the blood to move to a more distal location. Ischemic rest pain does not affect the calf muscles.

Appearance of Spectral Waveform

Any time a vascular technologist believes that a patient has a hemodynamically significant stenosis or occlusion of a peripheral artery, it is especially important to make sure that the Doppler parameters are set correctly. Of course, gray-scale, color, and spectral Doppler will be used to complete the ultrasound exam. If a patient has a hemodynamically significant stenosis of the leg, the waveform distal to the diseased artery likely demonstrates poststenotic turbulence and bidirectional flow may be seen as the blood is leaving the area of the blood vessel that is narrowed. Monophasic waveforms may also be present instead of the normal triphasic signals because the blood flow is not reversed. Some of the energy is lost because of the lesion, so there will be reduced peak velocities with the loss of the dicrotic notch.

Mesenteric Vasculature Disease

Celiac, Superior Mesenteric, and Inferior Mesenteric Arteries

The organs of digestion are fed by three main vessels: the celiac artery, the superior mesenteric artery (SMA), and the inferior mesenteric artery. In a patient presenting with intestinal ischemia, two out of the three blood vessels must demonstrate a significant stenosis with the SMA acting as the artery that supplies the majority of oxygenated blood to the intestines. Vascular technologists will not encounter chronic mesenteric ischemia very often, but when it is present, it develops from atherosclerotic disease. Another reason that chronic mesenteric ischemia is rare is because of the collateral channels that enable the blood to flow to the digestive organs. The arc of Riolan and gastroduodenal artery are two such vessels that keep blood flowing in the presence of a significant stenosis.

Symptoms of Diseased Mesenteric Arteries

Patients that have chronic mesenteric ischemia may experience nausea, vomiting, and diarrhea. Patients may experience weight loss because of the pain that is experienced when they eat, so they often avoid food. Postprandial pain is a common symptom of bowel ischemia, and it occurs after meals when there is more of a need for blood to reach the intestines. This is also known as bowel claudication because the symptoms arise after there is a need for an increased supply of blood or intestinal ischemia. An abdominal bruit may be present as well. Females are often at a higher risk of suffering from acute mesenteric ischemia, especially those women that are within the age group of 60 to 80 years old. Most cases of chronic mesenteric ischemia are due to significant stenosis of the SMA as well as either the celiac or inferior mesenteric artery.

Copyright © Mometrix Media. You have been licensed one copy of this document for personal use only. Any other reproduction or redistribution is strictly prohibited. All rights reserved.
This content is provided for test preparation purposes only and does not imply an endorsement by Mometrix of any particular political, scientific, or religious point of view.

Examining the Celiac Artery with Ultrasound vs. CTA

Before starting an exam, vascular technologists are taught to always look at previous exams and/or imaging reports for comparison. Sometimes there can be a discrepancy in the findings, especially if a patient has undergone computed tomography angiography (CTA) to evaluate the mesenteric blood vessels. For example, if a patient presents with symptoms of median arcuate ligament syndrome, the CTA may appear normal because the exam is done while the patient suspends respiration upon deep inspiration. Even if the patient is positive for median arcuate ligament syndrome, the CTA may appear normal because often the deep breath can create this situation. Ultrasound, however, can be performed when the patient is in quiet respiration, deep inspiration, and even during expiration. The vascular technologist has the ability to scan the patient while lying on their back and also in an upright position. Having the patient sit or stand up causes the celiac artery to drop down into the abdomen more, which can alleviate the confinement on the celiac artery caused by the median arcuate ligament.

Celiac Artery Compression Syndrome

Celiac artery compression syndrome occurs when the median arcuate ligament travels anterior to the celiac artery (instead of above the point at which the celiac artery arises from the abdominal aorta), which can create severe pain when the artery is compressed by the ligament. This pain is often postprandial and may be accompanied by nausea, diarrhea, and weight loss. Physicians may also hear a bruit in the epigastric region that may fluctuate with the patient's breathing. The pain may be caused by the compression of the nerves in the area of the celiac artery, or it could be due to the decreased perfusion to the digestive organs. Ultrasound can be used to examine the celiac axis in multiple patient positions, fasting states, and with various breathing techniques to determine the cause. If the PSV is more than 200 cm/s in the fasting state, it is highly suspicious for a significant stenosis or occlusion of the celiac artery. Celiac artery compression syndrome is also referred to as median arcuate ligament syndrome.

Renal Vasculature Disease

Typical Visualization of Atherosclerosis

Renal artery stenosis can stem from many conditions including atherosclerosis and thrombosis, embolism, and fibromuscular dysplasia. When a renal artery duplex exam is performed, the kidneys and abdominal aorta are also interrogated. When atherosclerosis is present in the renal arteries, it tends to be present in the proximal segment of the renal arteries where they branch from the abdominal aorta. If the mid and distal segments are diseased, it tends to be the result of fibromuscular dysplasia. Proximal renal artery stenosis can be assumed when the renal/aortic velocity ratio has been calculated as being greater than 3.5.

Nutcracker Syndrome

Nutcracker syndrome may include two variations, both of which compress the left renal vein. The left renal vein originates at the renal hilum and must cross the midline of the body to empty into the IVC, which lies to the right of the spine. On the

Copyright © Mometrix Media. You have been licensed one copy of this document for personal use only. Any other reproduction or redistribution is strictly prohibited. All rights reserved.
This content is provided for test preparation purposes only and does not imply an endorsement by Mometrix of any particular political, scientific, or religious point of view.

way to the IVC, the left renal vein passes in between the SMA and the abdominal aorta. When the blood within the left renal vein cannot flow normally because it is impeded by the SMA and/or the abdominal aorta, it becomes disrupted. If the left renal vein passes posterior to the abdominal aorta (referred to as the retroaortic left renal vein), it can also become compressed by the larger aorta, which can cause venous stasis.

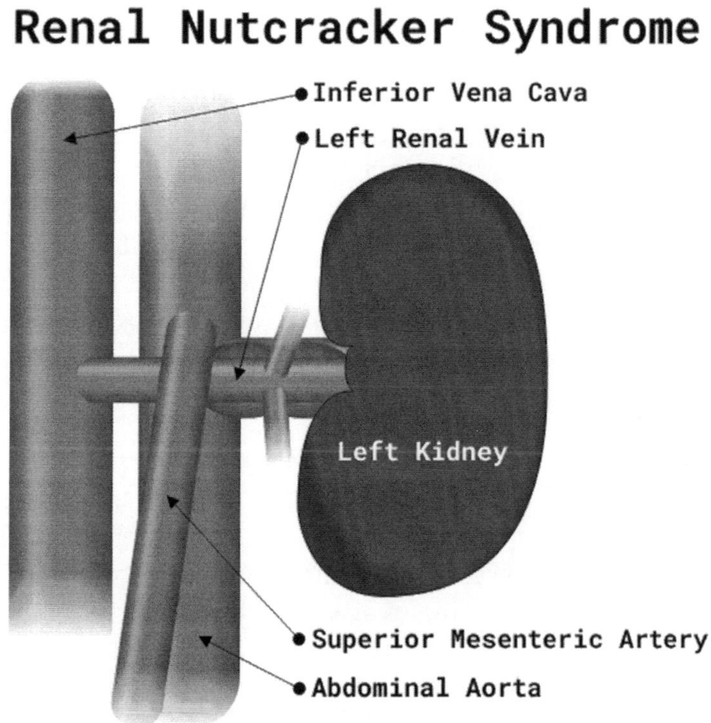

Common Congenital Anomaly of the Renal Artery

The renal arteries originate from the abdominal aorta and carry oxygenated blood to the kidneys. Typically, most patients have two kidneys (one on either side of the spine). These organs are supplied by the renal artery, and although most individuals only have one renal artery on each side, it is not uncommon to see more than one renal artery. In fact, the most common congenital anomaly of the renal artery is multiple arteries that supply the kidneys, which is seen in roughly 30% of people. This can occur unilaterally, and when it is unilateral, it seems to develop on either side with equal prevalence but can also be found bilaterally in the same patient. Just like patients that only have one renal artery per side, multiple arteries typically stem from the same region of the aorta in those patients. However, they may also arise from the superior or inferior mesenteric arteries or even the common iliacs. In patients with congenital variants of the urinary system such as horseshoe or ectopic kidneys, it is not uncommon to see variations where the renal arteries arise.

Renal Artery with Reversal of Flow During Diastole

The renal arteries have low-resistance flow because these blood vessels are carrying blood to the kidneys, which are extremely vascular organs. Spectral analysis will

Copyright © Mometrix Media. You have been licensed one copy of this document for personal use only. Any other reproduction or redistribution is strictly prohibited. All rights reserved.
This content is provided for test preparation purposes only and does not imply an endorsement by Mometrix of any particular political, scientific, or religious point of view.

demonstrate an arterial waveform of high resistance if the patient has kidney disease. A normal renal artery should also have an acceleration index of greater than 300 cm/s^2. If the waveform of the renal artery has a reversal of flow during diastole (which is not normal), the vascular technologist must carefully evaluate the ipsilateral renal vein. If there is a thrombus present in the renal vein, it could create outflow obstruction, which could cause the reversal of flow in diastole of the renal artery.

Renal/Aortic Ratio

Ultrasound is a useful and noninvasive modality to help diagnose renal artery stenosis. It is important to use a system that has the capability of providing gray-scale, color, and spectral Doppler functions to make sure that the correct vessel is being interrogated. One of the calculations that the ultrasound machine can provide is the renal/aortic ratio, which is a comparison of the highest PSV of the main renal artery to the aortic PSV. If the computed value of the systolic renal/aortic velocity is greater than 3.5, this suggests the possibility of a renal artery stenosis of 60% or more.

Primary and Secondary Hypertension

Hypertension can be placed in one of two categories: primary or secondary. Primary hypertension (also referred to as essential hypertension) is the category in which a large percentage of the population falls into (95%). There appears to be no single, definitive cause of primary hypertension; rather, there is a combination of factors such as insulin resistance, aging, being overweight, poor nutrition, not getting enough (or any) exercise, a long-term considerable amount of alcohol consumption, and genetics. Secondary hypertension is known as renovascular hypertension. This type of high blood pressure is caused by a coexisting disorder that is already affecting the heart, arteries, kidneys, or endocrine system, or it is even caused by drug abuse. Although a small percentage of patients have this type of hypertension, it is usually due to the development of atherosclerosis and is found in patients that are older than 50.

Evaluating the Renal Veins

The renal veins are responsible for returning blood that has been depleted of oxygen from the kidneys back to the heart. Typically, there is one renal vein for each kidney, but the ultrasound technologist may see more than one vessel on the same side. Renal veins empty the blood into the IVC so it can travel to the right atrium of the heart. The renal vein may develop a thrombus, especially if a clot is present in the IVC. Another condition of the renal veins that may be picked up during an ultrasound exam is a tumor invasion from a primary renal cell carcinoma. Vascular technologists should also evaluate the renal veins for possible compression of the left renal vein from the aorta or SMA as it travels between these two structures on the way to the IVC.

Copyright © Mometrix Media. You have been licensed one copy of this document for personal use only. Any other reproduction or redistribution is strictly prohibited. All rights reserved.
This content is provided for test preparation purposes only and does not imply an endorsement by Mometrix of any particular political, scientific, or religious point of view.

Horseshoe Kidneys

Horseshoe kidneys are the most common congenital fusion abnormality and are often an incidental diagnosis. People with horseshoe kidneys can lead a normal life, but it is important to diagnose horseshoe kidneys prior to any abdominal surgery because the anatomy can vary so it is important for the surgical team to be aware of this condition. Also, for anybody that needs renal imaging or procedures to be performed, it is imperative to be aware of this anomaly beforehand because it is not uncommon to have multiple renal arteries with horseshoe kidneys. A patient with horseshoe kidneys demonstrates a lower lying position of the kidneys that are positioned near the middle of the body. Horseshoe kidneys are typically fused at the lower poles, which tend to be directed in a more medial position. Although some individuals don't have any issues at all, others will be prone to kidney stones, hydronephrosis, or urinary tract infections. The diagram demonstrates horseshoe kidneys that are fused at the lower poles.

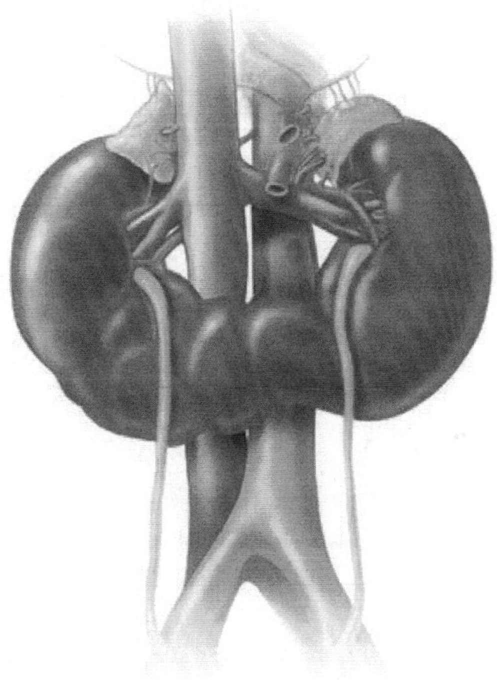

Hepatoportal System Disease

Portal Hypertension

The liver is an essential organ: One of its functions is to eliminate toxins from the body. The portal vein transports a large percentage of blood from the bowel to the liver. When the pressure inside the portal system is elevated more than 5 mmHg than the pressure within the IVC, it is referred to as portal hypertension (PHTN). PHTN can be caused by several factors, such as anatomical variations that can lead to an increase of pressure or liver disease. Elevated pressures may be due to obstruction of the portal venous system or hepatic veins. Cirrhosis is often

Copyright © Mometrix Media. You have been licensed one copy of this document for personal use only. Any other reproduction or redistribution is strictly prohibited. All rights reserved.
This content is provided for test preparation purposes only and does not imply an endorsement by Mometrix of any particular political, scientific, or religious point of view.

responsible for an increase in resistance because scarring of the liver tissue reduces blood flow to the liver and increases pressure within the venous portal system.

Sonographic Findings Suggesting PHTN

There are many conditions that cause PHTN such as cirrhosis, pancreatitis, blood clots, and cancer. When scanning the liver, vascular technologists will typically notice portosystemic venous collaterals on gray-scale and color Doppler images. The portal vein may appear enlarged with a diameter of at least 13 mm, or it may demonstrate portal vein thrombosis, splenomegaly, or ascites. Pulsed-wave and color Doppler may demonstrate hepatofugal flow, which means that the blood is traveling in the wrong direction and away from the liver instead of the normal hepatopetal flow that moves toward the liver from the bowel. Clinically, the patient may present with gastrointestinal bleeding and leg edema, and dilated veins may be visualized on the abdominal wall of the patient.

Budd-Chiari Syndrome

The blood within the liver is returned to the IVC via the right, middle, and left hepatic veins. Budd-Chiari syndrome is a condition in which thrombus is present within the hepatic veins. If these vessels are clotted, then the blood within the liver cannot be returned to the heart, which can lead to further problems such as PHTN. Gray-scale imaging will demonstrate filling defects within the hepatic vein(s). Collateral channels may be visualized along with splenomegaly and ascites. Color and spectral Doppler should be used as well to prove the absence of flow within these vessels. The patient's liver function tests will likely be higher than normal, and the patient may experience abdominal pain. Budd-Chiari syndrome may stem from tumor invasion or thrombus within the IVC, so it is important to carefully examine this structure.

Hepatofugal Blood Flow

The liver is one of the most vascular organs that humans have because of its dual blood supply. Not only does the hepatic artery carry oxygenated blood to the liver, but the portal venous system also transports blood into the liver from the digestive system. Hepatofugal flow is an abnormality of the direction of blood flow that takes place when flow patterns within the venous portal system move away from the liver instead of toward the liver. This occurs most commonly because of the pressure buildup in the portal system such as in the case of patients with cirrhosis, which will often result in PHTN. The diagnosis of hepatofugal flow is important to discern because it is often linked to a reduced survival outcome in patients with cirrhosis or patients that have had a liver transplant. The hepatic veins also demonstrate hepatofugal flow as they carry blood away from the liver and dump it into the IVC.

Life-Threatening Esophageal Varices

When the submucosal veins of the inferior portion of the esophagus become distended, it indicates that esophageal varices are present. This is a serious complication of PHTN because bleeding can occur, and if it isn't diagnosed and managed quickly, a significant amount of bleeding can occur. If these vessels

Copyright © Mometrix Media. You have been licensed one copy of this document for personal use only. Any other reproduction or redistribution is strictly prohibited. All rights reserved.
This content is provided for test preparation purposes only and does not imply an endorsement by Mometrix of any particular political, scientific, or religious point of view.

rupture, it can be deadly for the patient. In those with PHTN, the blood flowing into the liver is reduced. The coronary (gastric) vein will typically carry blood into the splenic vein (which joins the superior mesenteric vein to form the main portal vein). The veins that tend to empty into the portal system can no longer continue this function, so they end up dumping into the other vessels known as collateral channels. This rise in pressure causes the coronary vein blood to flow in the other direction, which creates esophageal varices.

Dilated Coronary Vein's Role in PHTN

Veins in the upper two-thirds of the esophagus return deoxygenated blood into the azygos vein, which eventually carries blood to the right atrium via the superior vena cava. These vessels do not play a role in the evolution of the dilated submucosal veins that are found in the inferior third portion of the esophagus known as esophageal varices. The coronary vein (also referred to as the left gastric vein) is a small vessel that has a diameter of about 1 mm. When this vein becomes dilated due to PHTN, it can reach a diameter of 1–2 cm, which can cause severe bleeding and even death. The coronary vein transports blood to the portal vein, but if PHTN is present, the direction of blood flow may reverse and end up emptying into the collateral varices instead.

Examining the Hepatic Veins During

Three hepatic veins are present within the liver; these are the right, middle, and left hepatic veins. These blood vessels remove deoxygenated blood from the liver by emptying the blood into the IVC to be returned to the right atrium of the heart. If the blood within the liver cannot be properly routed to the IVC, congestion of the liver can take place. This surplus of blood can impede liver function and cause PHTN. During a scenario such as this, PHTN is the result of a rise in pressure of the portal system when the hepatic veins are clotted. Tumor invasion can also be the cause of PHTN, so it is important to examine as much of the IVC in addition to the hepatic veins during an abdominal ultrasound.

Rayleigh Scattering During an Exam

Scattering is an erratic, unsystematic diversion of the ultrasound beam in multiple directions. Rayleigh scattering is just one type of scattering, but instead of being erratic, the sound wave is directed in 360 degrees in an organized manner. Rayleigh scattering takes place because the actual size of the target is much smaller than the wavelength of the ultrasound beam. For example, if a vascular technologist can visualize blood flow in hepatic vessels without color-flow Doppler, it is due to Rayleigh scattering. The red blood cells are the target of the ultrasound system, but the image may be misinterpreted because without color flow the vessels may appear as if they are clotted. If the user decreases the frequency, then the signal amplitude of what may appear as a clot in the hepatic vessels should be less apparent. Rayleigh scattering is proportional to the frequency to the fourth power.

Copyright © Mometrix Media. You have been licensed one copy of this document for personal use only. Any other reproduction or redistribution is strictly prohibited. All rights reserved.
This content is provided for test preparation purposes only and does not imply an endorsement by Mometrix of any particular political, scientific, or religious point of view.

Paraumbilical Vein

The paraumbilical vein starts at the umbilicus and travels between the layers of the falciform ligament and continues into the left portal vein. When visualized sonographically, it will have an anechoic and tubular configuration connecting the umbilicus to the falciform ligament. This blood vessel is important during pregnancy because it facilitates the transportation of oxygenated blood from the placenta and carries it to the liver of the developing fetus via the umbilical cord. Ultrasound imaging of the paraumbilical vein is not usually possible because this blood vessel is not usually evident with sonography, even in the pediatric population. However, this blood vessel may become enlarged in individuals that have PHTN so that the pressure within the portal veins can be reduced when these channels recanalize so the blood in the paraumbilical vein can move the blood into the superficial epigastric vein. This vessel may recanalize in patients that have cirrhosis as well.

IVC and/or Iliac Vein Disease

Using Shallow Breathing in the Ultrasound Study

When the IVC is of interest, it should be evaluated with gray-scale, color, and pulsed-wave Doppler by using a curvilinear transducer. An exhaustive scan of the liver should also be completed in addition to the hepatic veins. The hepatic veins return blood from the liver into the IVC. If a blood clot is present within the IVC, it should be seen with gray-scale imaging. In addition, the ultrasound user should also evaluate with color and spectral Doppler because these methods can provide additional information within the blood vessel as well as gather waveforms. The IVC and hepatic veins should be studied when the patient is breathing normally because deep breaths will compress the IVC and cause the forward flow to stop momentarily. The normal waveform of the IVC should demonstrate pulsatility due to the close proximity to the heart. If this pulsatility is absent or the waveform appears dampened, then a central IVC obstruction is possible.

Scenario

While using gray-scale ultrasound, a blood clot is visualized in the IVC. Explain why this clot will reach the right atrium prior to any other chamber of the heart.

Arteries are the vessels that carry oxygenated blood to all cells in the body. Once the cells have taken from the blood the nutrients and oxygen that they need, the blood is returned to the right side of the heart before reaching the lungs to pick up oxygen once again. Blood that has been depleted of oxygen from the level above the heart is emptied into the SVC, which dumps blood into the right atrium of the heart. Blood is returned from the level below the heart from the IVC, which also empties into the right atrium. If a clot is present in the IVC and it breaks off, it will first travel to the right atrium, which is the first of the four chambers of the heart that blood travels in.

Extracranial Cerebrovascular Disease

Appearance of the Waveform in the Right CCA

A carotid duplex ultrasound exam is a reliable, noninvasive exam used to determine the patency and direction of blood flow within various arteries. Spectral Doppler is

Copyright © Mometrix Media. You have been licensed one copy of this document for personal use only. Any other reproduction or redistribution is strictly prohibited. All rights reserved.
This content is provided for test preparation purposes only and does not imply an endorsement by Mometrix of any particular political, scientific, or religious point of view.

an important component of a carotid duplex exam because each artery has a typical appearance (which will fluctuate a bit based on each patient that is examined) based on which organs and tissues are being supplied. For example, the CCA will demonstrate diastolic flow of moderate proportions and low-resistance flow as the majority of the blood continues into the ICA, which feeds the brain. When a distal occlusion is present and the right ICA is occluded, there will be less diastolic flow, which is created when there is more resistance. If the right ICA is completely occluded, then it would not be surprising to see an absence of flow within the right CCA.

Subclavian Steal Syndrome

The vertebral arteries are a conduit for blood flow to the brain. In cases of a subclavian steal, the blood travels to the arm instead of the brain on the affected side. This is due to a stenosis or even total occlusion in a location that is proximal to the vertebral artery (such as in the innominate or subclavian artery). The origin of the left subclavian artery is the aortic arch, so this is a condition that is seen more often on the left side. If the blood pressure is measured on both arms, the systolic component of the affected side is at least 15–20 mmHg less than the other side. Ultrasound will demonstrate a reversal of flow in the ipsilateral vertebral artery if there is complete occlusion of the subclavian artery. If the proximal vessels are not completely occluded, then the waveforms can vary depending on the amount of stenosis and can vary from early systolic deceleration to bidirectional flow as the stenosis becomes more advanced. The diagram demonstrates the blood from the right vertebral artery moving into the left vertebral artery to help supply the left arm because the proximal left subclavian artery is occluded.

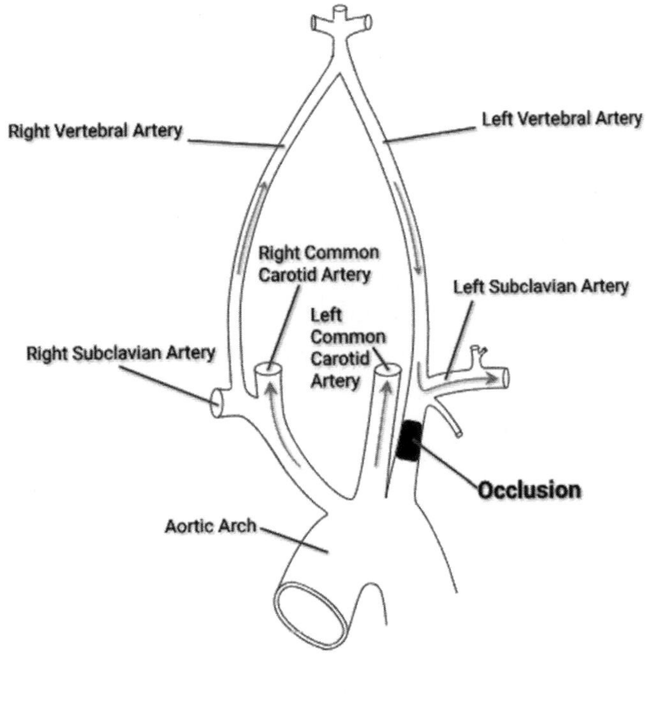

Copyright © Mometrix Media. You have been licensed one copy of this document for personal use only. Any other reproduction or redistribution is strictly prohibited. All rights reserved.
This content is provided for test preparation purposes only and does not imply an endorsement by Mometrix of any particular political, scientific, or religious point of view.

Takayasu's Arteritis

Takayasu's arteritis is a condition in which the walls of the aorta and its branches become thickened due to inflammation. This thickening of the arterial walls eventually leads to vessels that are stenotic and that may become occluded over time. One of the main symptoms of this disorder is a reduced or even a complete inability to find a pulse in the patient's extremities. Other symptoms are dizziness, vertigo, headaches, and hypertension, and even heart attacks and strokes have been reported. This condition is rare and is typically seen in women that are younger than 40 (and in some cases even in their teenage years) and is believed to be an autoimmune disorder. The narrowed vessels may be seen in gray-scale ultrasound imaging, but angiography is the modality that is used most often to make an accurate diagnosis of Takayasu's arteritis.

Scenarios for Turbulent Blood Flow

The type of blood flow that makes up the majority of flow dynamics within the blood vessels of the human body is known as laminar flow. During laminar flow, red blood cells within the center of the vessel are moving faster than those in the outer walls in a more layered appearance. Turbulence is considered to be flow that is not orderly or layered such as that found in laminar flow. Turbulent flow is often noted distal to a segment of vessel that is stenotic, but this type of blood flow is also evident in blood vessels that are not diseased and may even be considered normal in some arteries. Turbulent flow may be noticed in patients that have vessels that are tortuous or when the artery is kinked. Turbulence may also be witnessed when the artery becomes expanded, such as in the region of the carotid bulb.

Scenario

During a carotid duplex study, if color flow demonstrates blood flow in the carotid bulb but not the ICA, discuss what the vascular technologist may assume and how to continue the exam.

During a carotid duplex study, if the vascular technologist can obtain color flow in the carotid bulb, but not in the ICA, then it should be assumed that the ICA is totally occluded. However, it is important to continue the exam by using continuous-wave and/or pulsed-wave Doppler in addition to gray-scale, color, and power Doppler. The vascular technologist should make several attempts to determine flow because the patient is managed differently depending on whether the diagnosis is total or occlusion or a critical stenosis. Patients with a severe stenosis may be candidates for a carotid endarterectomy, but this is not the case when the ICA is totally occluded. Ultrasound is often the first study performed if carotid artery disease is suspected, but it may be followed up with a magnetic resonance angiogram or a carotid angiogram, which is a more invasive test.

Amaurosis Fugax

The ophthalmic artery is the first branch of the ICA and is extremely important because it and all of its branches supplies the eye with the necessary blood flow. If a patient has ulcerated plaque within their ICA, one of the risks is a thromboembolic

Copyright © Mometrix Media. You have been licensed one copy of this document for personal use only. Any other reproduction or redistribution is strictly prohibited. All rights reserved.
This content is provided for test preparation purposes only and does not imply an endorsement by Mometrix of any particular political, scientific, or religious point of view.

event that can create the effect of a shade that has dropped down over the eye or part of the eye and interferes with the patient's vision. This blindness that the patient experiences is temporary (often lasting 30 minutes or less), and the affected ophthalmic artery is on the same side as the diseased ICA in which the embolus traveled from and is characterized as a monocular episode.

Typical Location of Atherosclerosis

Atherosclerosis is a disease that progresses over time and is one of the leading causes of strokes and heart attacks. With this condition, plaque tends to create a narrowing of the blood vessels, which can limit the amount of blood flow to vital organs. Plaque is the result of a buildup of fat and cholesterol in an artery that can create a thickening of the intima of the arterial wall. Sometimes, this thickening extends into the middle layer in addition to the inner layer. This accumulation of plaque can create a narrowing of the artery known as stenosis. During a carotid duplex exam, the vascular technologist will often locate atherosclerosis at the bifurcation of the carotid artery, especially where the ICA branches from the CCA.

Cerebrovascular Accident

A cerebrovascular accident (CVA) is the medical term for a stroke, which is a medical emergency. A stroke occurs because of an interruption of blood flow to the brain or if a blood vessel ruptures. Ischemic strokes are the most common type (approximately 85%), which happens when a blood clot forms in an artery that supplies the brain with blood (referred to as a thrombotic stroke). Another cause of an ischemic stroke is when a thrombus organizes in a different part of the body but breaks off and ends up in a smaller artery within the brain (known as an embolic stroke). The other 15% of strokes are hemorrhagic in nature, which may be from an aneurysm or other cause of bleeding in the brain. Although occurring less often, hemorrhagic strokes are often fatal.

Inaccurate Measurements from a Pulsed-Wave Doppler

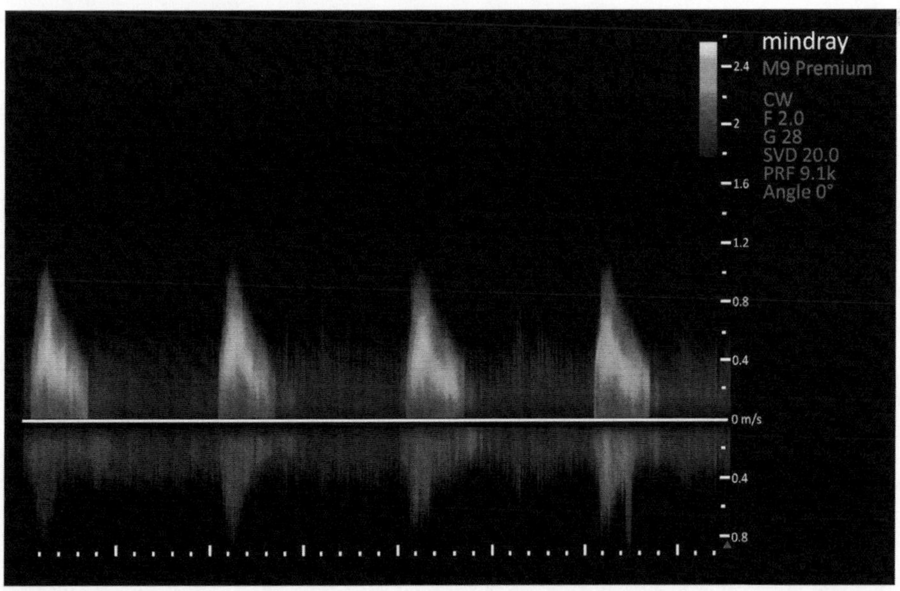

Copyright © Mometrix Media. You have been licensed one copy of this document for personal use only. Any other reproduction or redistribution is strictly prohibited. All rights reserved.
This content is provided for test preparation purposes only and does not imply an endorsement by Mometrix of any particular political, scientific, or religious point of view.

Pulsed-wave Doppler is a useful method to measure blood flow velocities within various blood vessels. The ultrasound user has the option to select where the gate should be placed within a vessel in order to take a velocity measurement and know the exact location of this reading. However, sometimes, the velocity within the blood vessel is too high and the sonographer is unable to obtain an accurate peak velocity measurement. The sonographer would want to switch to continuous-wave Doppler because velocities that are extremely high tend to be more accurate because there isn't a maximum velocity while using this method. While using pulsed-wave Doppler, if the user cannot eliminate aliasing after trying to change the scale, the depth of the target, and switching to a lower frequency probe, then he or she can switch to continuous-wave Doppler.

Carotid Dissection

A carotid dissection occurs when the tunica intima (inner) layer of the arterial wall is torn, which enables blood to get between the layers of the arterial wall. Much like an aortic dissection, a false lumen develops and can expand in both directions, which may cause an obstruction. The sonographic visualization of an intimal flap in the carotid artery can help diagnose a carotid dissection. It is important to note that the blood within the false lumen may clot or even embolize, which can lead to a stroke. Color and spectral Doppler may demonstrate blood flowing in opposite directions in the false and true lumens. Spectral Doppler signals may also show different velocities on either side of the intimal flap. Carotid dissections are typically the result of trauma such as a motorcycle or car accident, especially in the younger population. Spontaneous dissections have been reported, although they are not as common. Individuals with connective tissue disorders such as Marfan syndrome or Ehlers-Danlos syndrome are at a slightly higher risk of a dissection.

Types and Appearances of Atherosclerotic Plaque

During a carotid duplex exam, vascular technologists will encounter various types and appearances of atherosclerotic plaque within the carotid arteries. Clinicians can use ultrasound as a predictive tool to help determine individuals that have the greatest risk of a stroke by evaluating who has plaque that appears suspicious for hemorrhage or ulceration. If the lesion contains plaque that consists of fibrous tissue, calcium, cellular particles, and collagen, it is referred to as a complicated lesion, which often takes on a heterogenous appearance. An ulcerative plaque is especially concerning because particles may break off and become lodged in a distal artery causing a transient ischemic attack, or stroke. This is considered an unstable plaque because the surface of the lesion begins to break down to allow the contents within to possibly escape. An intraplaque hemorrhage is identified when a low-level echogenic component is seen within a plaque. This condition also puts the patient at a greater risk of embolism if there is a rupture.

Carotid Endarterectomy

A carotid endarterectomy is a procedure in which the surgeon exposes the lumen of the carotid artery in order to visualize and remove plaque that has accumulated within the vessel. This procedure is performed to reduce the risk of an ischemic

Copyright © Mometrix Media. You have been licensed one copy of this document for personal use only. Any other reproduction or redistribution is strictly prohibited. All rights reserved.
This content is provided for test preparation purposes only and does not imply an endorsement by Mometrix of any particular political, scientific, or religious point of view.

stroke. Often, patients present to the ultrasound lab not because they are symptomatic, but rather their physician detected a carotid bruit, which suggests carotid stenosis. Other patients describe transient ischemic attack symptoms such as a temporary loss of vision, speech, weakness, or numbness that occurs unilaterally. Patients that undergo this type of surgery must be watched closely for complications such as breathing issues if the trachea is compressed by a hematoma that has developed, bleeding of the incision, or neointimal hyperplasia. Neointimal hyperplasia is often responsible for restenosis between 6 and 24 months postoperative because there is rapid growth of the smooth muscle cells as the tissue is attempting to heal. Notably, this procedure is not performed when a complete occlusion of the ICA has been proven.

Abnormal Sound in the Neck

When a healthcare provider uses the stethoscope to listen to a patient's neck and hears an abnormal sound, it is referred to as a bruit. Laminar flow is the typical blood flow pattern, but a bruit that occurs when this pattern is no longer present is often the result of turbulent blood flow such as in the case of a carotid stenosis. However, providers must not rely on the presence or absence of an audible bruit to diagnose disease. If a bruit is heard and it continues in diastole, the provider will be especially concerned because this is indicative of a significant stenosis of 70%–80% lumen diameter reduction. If a bruit was previously heard in a patient but is no longer present, this likely means that the diameter reduction is now more than 90% and the disease classification is now considered to be preocclusive.

Obtaining Reliable Measurement of the PSV

Often during a carotid duplex exam, a vascular technologist will notice an incidental cardiac arrhythmia on a patient. This does not typically pose a problem during the exam, and it is possible to obtain a reliable measurement of the PSV once the sinus rhythm becomes normal again. Ultrasound protocols may vary from one lab to another in patients that have a severe cardiac arrhythmia because attaining PSV measurements can often be difficult. It may be advantageous to obtain a ratio of the highest measured PSV of the ICA and compare it to the distal CCA PSV. Interpreting physicians may request that the vascular technologist averages 3 or 4 cycles (although some will require up to 10 cycles) as the preferred protocol in cases of severe arrhythmias.

Intracranial Cerebrovascular Disease

Abnormality Visualized in the Circle of Willis

The circle of Willis is an arterial ring that is comprised of segments of the anterior and posterior intracranial blood vessels. This structure is about the same diameter of a 50-cent piece and sits at the base of the brain. The blood vessels that are part of the circle of Willis are the distal internal carotid, anterior cerebral, posterior cerebral, and communicating arteries. Although the name suggests that this connection is complete, less than 50% of the population has a circle of Willis that is fully developed. One of the most common abnormalities of this structure is the lack of at least one of the two communicating arteries. Having a circle of Willis that is

Copyright © Mometrix Media. You have been licensed one copy of this document for personal use only. Any other reproduction or redistribution is strictly prohibited. All rights reserved.
This content is provided for test preparation purposes only and does not imply an endorsement by Mometrix of any particular political, scientific, or religious point of view.

fully developed is advantageous if the patient develops a significant stenosis or blockage and it can serve as a collateral channel.

Occluded Artery When a CVA Occurs

A CVA is an interruption of blood flow to the brain either due to an occlusion or a rupture of a blood vessel such as an aneurysm. The MCA is the cerebral artery that is occluded more than others to cause a stroke, otherwise known as a large-vessel stroke. The MCA stems from the ICA and takes a more lateral direction to supply the temporal, parietal, and frontal lobes of the brain with oxygenated blood. A CVA caused by the occlusion (or a possible bleed) of the MCA may result in numbness on the contralateral side of the body of the patient. Hemiplegia is also another symptom that the individual may experience.

Vasospasm and Typical Findings

A vasospasm causes the arteries in the body to contract, which greatly diminishes the amount of blood flow to the organs. Vasospasms can happen in all regions of the body, but when they occur in the brain, it is often the result of a ruptured brain aneurysm that created a subarachnoid hemorrhage. This hemorrhaging causes the arteries within the brain to contract; often, a couple of days later the complication of vasospasm sets in. TCD can be used to evaluate the velocity of the cerebral arteries and determine if vasospasm is present. A higher velocity within the cerebral arteries equals a greater chance of brain damage. Vasospasm usually maxes out around one to two weeks after the subarachnoid hemorrhage occurred and is noticeable in the cerebral arteries that are more prominent such as the MCA.

Temporal Arteritis

Vasculitis can be defined as the swelling of blood vessels. Temporal arteritis is one kind of vasculitis that occurs when the distal portion of the superficial temporal artery becomes inflamed. The external carotid arteries give rise to the temporal vessels, which are found near the temples of the patient and supply the scalp with oxygenated blood. The temporal artery divides into the frontal and parietal branches, which may also be affected. Although this is an extremely difficult diagnosis to make with ultrasound, the vessel will appear narrowed and edema may surround the lumen of the artery on gray-scale and color Doppler imaging. This condition is often diagnosed in women that are older than age 50; it is important to diagnose temporal arteritis quickly because the patient's vision may be lost if the arteries that supply blood to the eye are also affected.

Incidental Findings

Carotid Body Tumor

A carotid body tumor is a rare finding that may be visualized when a vascular technologist is performing a carotid duplex exam on a patient or if the patient presents with a palpable neck mass. If a mass is identified that demonstrates an extreme amount of vascularity and is situated between the ECA and the ICA, then the vascular technologist should suspect a carotid body tumor. These masses are typically supplied with blood from the ECA and tend to grow slowly, but over time

Copyright © Mometrix Media. You have been licensed one copy of this document for personal use only. Any other reproduction or redistribution is strictly prohibited. All rights reserved.
This content is provided for test preparation purposes only and does not imply an endorsement by Mometrix of any particular political, scientific, or religious point of view.

they can develop into a prominent mass. The patient may notice a pulsatile mass in the upper region of the neck, difficulty swallowing, neck and shoulder pain, as well as modifications in vision and blood pressure. Typically, symptoms do not manifest until the tumor becomes sizable. Although rarely cancerous, treatment of carotid body tumors includes radiation therapy, surgical excision, and embolization.

Baker's Cyst

Synovial fluid is found in joint capsules, and it aids in the reduction of friction when an individual uses his or her limbs. If there is too much synovial fluid in the posterior knee, it is referred to as a Baker's cyst. This fluid collection will appear as a well-defined cystic component in the posterior and/or medial region within the popliteal fossa. Sometimes the patient may complain of a fullness behind their knee as well as pain, but often a Baker's cyst is an incidental finding without any symptoms. These fluid collections can occur because of an injury or because of inflammation associated with arthritis. These cysts may rupture, which occurs more often in patients who have osteoarthritis, gout, or in the elderly. During an ultrasound exam, a Baker's cyst that has ruptured will have a point as the fluid moves distally between the gastrocnemius and soleus muscles. The neck of this structure will be found between the semimembranosus tendon and the medial head of the gastrocnemius muscle.

Appearance of an Enlarged Lymph Node

During various ultrasound exams, a vascular technologist may discover enlarged lymph nodes throughout the body. These lymph nodes are often visualized in the neck, axilla, and groin and may be an incidental finding. Enlarged lymph nodes may be related to cancers such as lymphoma or to inflammation within the body. A normal lymph node takes on an oval or elliptical shape with a central hilum that is hyperechoic. A hypoechoic area will surround the hilum. When using color Doppler, the hilum will demonstrate some blood flow, but in a lymph node that is enlarged there is a lot of blood flow and the node itself tends to take on a more circular shape.

Masses

It is not uncommon for a vascular technologist to visualize masses in the neck while performing a carotid duplex study. For example, the patient may have enlarged lymph nodes that are apparent, especially if the patient has been sick recently. Medial to the carotid arteries is the thyroid gland, which is a butterfly-shaped gland located in the middle of the neck. It is not uncommon to find solid and cystic masses. Cysts contain fluid and are typically benign. Multinodular goiters are another common finding of the thyroid gland, which creates an enlarged thyroid. Nodules can be inflammatory if the patient has Hashimoto's disease, and other solid nodules may be present as well. Large masses can quickly be measured and documented as an incidental finding.

Venous Aneurysm

A venous aneurysm is a dilation of a vein that is 1.5 times larger than the adjacent segments of the same vessel. Venous aneurysms are not very common, but when

Copyright © Mometrix Media. You have been licensed one copy of this document for personal use only. Any other reproduction or redistribution is strictly prohibited. All rights reserved.
This content is provided for test preparation purposes only and does not imply an endorsement by Mometrix of any particular political, scientific, or religious point of view.

seen they may affect men or women of any age. They typically involve the veins of the legs and, more specifically, the popliteal vein, but they may occur in the jugular and upper extremities as well. Venous aneurysms may include complications such as blood clots or emboli, especially those that are diagnosed in the deep veins. Most individuals with a venous aneurysm complain of pain, swelling, and a palpable mass if the deep system is involved. If present in the groin region, they may be difficult to diagnose correctly without imaging because the symptoms are similar to those of a hernia. Surgery is often the course of action when a venous aneurysm is found.

Critical Findings

Virchow's Triad

In patients that have acquired a DVT, at least one of three risk factors must have taken place. Collectively, these circumstances are known as Virchow's triad. The first possible component is trauma, which could include something as simple as the placement of an IV or a blood draw that injures the wall of the vein. The second risk factor is stasis, which occurs when blood moves through the body more slowly than normal. Stasis can occur when a patient is bedridden or travels long distances while sitting, such as a long plane ride. Any time the blood starts to circulate at a slower pace or stop, a DVT is more likely to occur. The third component is hypercoagulability, which can be inherited, as is the case of factor V Leiden, acquired in individuals with cancer or women who use certain birth control methods, such as pills, rings, or patches.

Ultrasound and Clinical Findings

Patients that present to the vascular lab with a positive diagnosis of an acute DVT often complain of pain, swelling, and redness of the affected extremity. They may also complain of the extremity being warm to the touch. In situations in which the blood clot has traveled to the lungs, the patient may also explain symptoms of crushing chest pain and shortness of breath. Ultrasound findings of an acute DVT include the inability to completely compress the lumen of the affected vein(s). Gray-scale imaging will also demonstrate homogenous, low-level filling defects inside the vein that do not appear to adhere to the walls. Often, veins that are thrombosed will appear larger than normal. Color Doppler will not demonstrate complete filling of the vessel.

Flow Patterns in Arteries with a Significant Stenosis

An artery that exhibits a significant stenosis typically presents predictable flow patterns that vascular technologists are familiar with when performing ultrasound exams. In the area of the artery proximal to the stenotic lesion, it is common to see diminished blood flow velocities that may or may not be moving chaotically. As the blood travels through the area of the artery that is narrowed, increased velocities will be noted. Normal flow now becomes disorganized due to the formation of eddy currents. In the segment of the artery distal to the stenosis, turbulence is commonly present. As the artery becomes wider, flow separation takes place at the arterial walls. Bidirectional blood flow is common in the area of poststenotic turbulence, but

Copyright © Mometrix Media. You have been licensed one copy of this document for personal use only. Any other reproduction or redistribution is strictly prohibited. All rights reserved.
This content is provided for test preparation purposes only and does not imply an endorsement by Mometrix of any particular political, scientific, or religious point of view.

the velocity will be less than what was measured in the constricted portion of the artery.

Factors of Hemodynamically Stenosis

A stenotic lesion often turns into a hemodynamically stenosis when the diameter of the artery is reduced by half of the total for that vessel. The resulting area of the vessel would be 25% of the original cross section. A hemodynamically significant stenosis not only reduces the volume of blood flow, but also the pressure of the blood flowing. Other factors that influence if it will be a hemodynamically significant stenosis is how long the lesion is, the extensiveness of the stenosis, the shape that is formed from the lesion, the amount or presence of resistance that exists distal to the stenosis in the peripheral system, the texture of the surface of the arterial wall, and whether collateral channels are open for blood to pass through them.

Compartment Syndrome

Compartment syndrome is usually a diagnosis that is made clinically after an injury to the arms, legs, or less often the abdomen, and pressures within the compartment may be requested. The patient often presents with pain, swelling, muscle weakness, and numbness, and for cases that are more advanced it may be difficult to establish pulses in the extremity because they have become weakened or are not present. These symptoms are created due to bleeding that is associated with a great deal of swelling that occurs in the osteofascial compartments of the affected extremity. When this type of swelling develops, extrinsic compression reduces the blood flow so it can no longer reach the nerves or tissues and the muscle is at an increased risk of dying. Whether the case is acute or chronic, treatment includes a procedure called a fasciotomy, in which the contents of the compartment are cut open to allow for the swelling to dissipate.

Copyright © Mometrix Media. You have been licensed one copy of this document for personal use only. Any other reproduction or redistribution is strictly prohibited. All rights reserved.
This content is provided for test preparation purposes only and does not imply an endorsement by Mometrix of any particular political, scientific, or religious point of view.

Surgically Altered Anatomy and Pathology

Dialysis Access: Ability to Evaluate Postprocedural Vasculature

Placement of a TIPS

A transjugular intrahepatic portosystemic shunt (TIPS) is a low-resistance conduit that is created to establish a connection between the right branch of the portal vein and the hepatic vein. This procedure is performed under fluoroscopy by an interventional radiologist. The right jugular vein is the preferred access site to reach the hepatic vein because the liver is accessed from the superior and inferior vena cava. Once the catheter is within the hepatic vein, the pressure gradient in the liver is measured to help determine the extent of PHTN. TIPS is a highly successful therapeutic procedure for patients with cirrhosis who have developed PHTN or esophageal varices, and some individuals with ascites have had success with this kind of treatment.

Use of an IVC Filter

An IVC filter is a device that is used for patients diagnosed with DVT of the veins within the pelvis or lower legs. Candidates for IVC filters have a history of blood clots but are unable to undergo anticoagulation therapy (blood thinners). These individuals are at an especially high risk of developing a PE, in which a blood clot breaks off and moves toward the heart and blocks the pulmonary artery, which could be fatal for the patient. Initially, IVC interruption devices were considered permanent devices, but today these medical devices can be removed if necessary or can even be put in place as a temporary solution for individuals having a surgery that puts them at a higher risk of developing a blood clot.

Placement of an IVC Filter

The IVC filter is a medical device that is used to capture and trap any blood clots that may have traveled from the pelvis or lower extremities to prevent them from reaching the heart and/or lungs. There are several vendors that manufacture vena cava interruption devices, and they are produced in various shapes (often shaped like a cone) and sizes, but they are metal filters that are inserted into the IVC at a level that is located slightly below the point at which the renal veins enter this structure. IVC filters are placed by either interventional radiologists or vascular surgeons by inserting a catheter (which contains a flat IVC filter) into the patient's groin or neck, which is fed into the IVC. Once the catheter is extracted, the filter remains in place and will open up to become fixated to the IVC vessel wall.

Treatment Options for Risk of Losing a Leg

In the majority of patients that have been diagnosed with a DVT, the patient is able to undergo anticoagulation therapy in order to treat the blood clot. Although these blood thinners do not dissolve the clot, their purpose is to prevent the clot from breaking off or becoming bigger. Thrombolytics may be necessary for some patients

Copyright © Mometrix Media. You have been licensed one copy of this document for personal use only. Any other reproduction or redistribution is strictly prohibited. All rights reserved.
This content is provided for test preparation purposes only and does not imply an endorsement by Mometrix of any particular political, scientific, or religious point of view.

that are not responding well to the current blood thinner or who have developed pulmonary emboli. However, in some individuals the blood clot may be so extensive that even thrombolytic drugs won't work, especially if the iliofemoral portions are involved. In these cases, an iliofemoral venous thrombectomy may be the patient's best option to reduce complications such as the need to amputate the extremity, especially if it is treated early. New technology for a venous thrombectomy have improved the outcomes for the patient with fewer complications and significantly higher postprocedure patency rates without compromising valvular activity.

Access Method for Dialysis

For individuals that will undergo dialysis, the access method that is preferred would be an arteriovenous fistula (AVF) of the nondominant forearm. If the forearm can be used, the connection that is favored is the brachial artery to cephalic vein route. The forearm is favored over the upper arm, but if the nondominant forearm cannot be used, then the dominant forearm may be the site of access. Sonographic evaluation of the AVF includes measuring the diameter of the fistula as well as the draining vein (this should be 4 mm or more) to help determine if narrowing of these structures has occurred. A PSV ratio of 2:1 results in at least a 50% stenosis of the AVF when the draining vein is compared to a point 2 cm upstream.

Radiofrequency Ablation vs. Endovenous Laser Ablation

When the clinical management of varicose veins is not successful, venous ablation is a treatment option. When patients have an incompetent GSV or SSV, varicose veins are often the result and venous ablation has been successful to ease painful symptoms. There is little difference between the types of venous ablation. Radiofrequency ablation is one type of treatment option that uses an electrode to impart radiofrequency energy on the wall of the veins in order to create closure of the vein as the heat makes the collagen within the vessel contract. This technique tends to create less postprocedure pain and bruising. Endovenous laser ablation is a venous ablation technique that enables users a more controlled use of heat due to the use of a tiny optic laser that closes the vein due to the contraction of the wall. This is the preferred method if small clots are present or if the vein has a larger diameter.

Post Intervention

Use of Angle Correction During Spectral Doppler

Many venous flow studies do not require angle correction because the peak-systolic velocities (PSVs) are not measured. However, when evaluating a patient that has a transjugular intrahepatic portosystemic shunt (TIPS), it is imperative for the vascular technologist to use angle correction during the spectral Doppler portions of the exam because the PSVs must be measured. Protocols after a TIPS procedure include using color Doppler of the portal vein to check the direction of the blood flow and for signs of thrombus or occlusion. Spectral Doppler includes measuring PSVs in the segments of the portal vein that supplies blood to the TIPS, and the proximal, mid, and distal regions of the TIPS. It is also important to measure blood

Copyright © Mometrix Media. You have been licensed one copy of this document for personal use only. Any other reproduction or redistribution is strictly prohibited. All rights reserved.
This content is provided for test preparation purposes only and does not imply an endorsement by Mometrix of any particular political, scientific, or religious point of view.

flow distal to the TIPS in the hepatic vein. These PSVs should be measured with angle correction in mind, and the angle should be equal to or less than 60 degrees.

Complications Incurred During TIPS Insertion

Following TIPS insertion, complications may occur even though there have been high overall success rates because this is a very technical procedure to complete. It is important for the patient to have labs and a complete abdominal ultrasound workup prior to TIPS insertion to establish a baseline and to prevent complications. One of the most serious postprocedure complications is acute liver failure. Fortunately, this does not occur very often, but when it does happen, it is associated with a poor outcome for the patient unless a liver transplant is performed. Another rare complication is hemorrhaging during a TIPS procedure. Symptoms that the patient may have are abdominal pain and distension, vomiting blood, or abnormal blood pressure. Various injuries of arteries have also been reported, which may result in the occlusion of the artery or formation of a pseudoaneurysm.

Color Doppler Exam and Postablation Workups

A vascular technologist may be required to perform a color Doppler exam of the lower extremity immediately afterward as part of the postablation workup to confirm that the GSV has been thrombosed accordingly, which will be confirmed if there is not color flow within the GSV in the region of the SFJ. The vascular technologist should also check the superficial epigastric branch in addition to the femoral vein to make sure that these vessels are patent and to evaluate for possible extension of the superficial venous thrombosis into the deep venous system.

Myointimal Hyperplasia

Myointimal hyperplasia is concerning for an individual that has had a lower extremity bypass surgery performed because when stenosis develops in the first two years after the creation of a bypass graft it usually does so because of this condition. The area of the valve site is the typical location for the formation of stenosis. Myointimal hyperplasia can have a negative effect after bypass surgery because it can cause a blockage. Myointimal hyperplasia is the result of trauma to the endothelial cells after a grafting has taken place in which cells from the middle layer of the wall move to the inner layer and multiply and create a buildup when mixed with extracellular matrix, lymphocytes, and macrophages. This proliferation of cells can become problematic and lead to the constriction of the lumen of the blood vessel and hamper blood flow.

Aortobifemoral Bypass Graft

A bypass graft acts as a conduit that gives blood a different route to avoid an occlusion or serious stenosis. The purpose of a lower extremity bypass graft is to carry oxygenated blood around the lesion(s) within the artery that is (are) obstructing blood flow. This conduit must connect the region of the artery above the stenosis or occlusion with a region that is located below the area of the stenosis or occlusion in order to reestablish blood flow to both legs, which requires patent vessels in the proximal and distal locations. An aortobifemoral bypass graft is

Copyright © Mometrix Media. You have been licensed one copy of this document for personal use only. Any other reproduction or redistribution is strictly prohibited. All rights reserved.
This content is provided for test preparation purposes only and does not imply an endorsement by Mometrix of any particular political, scientific, or religious point of view.

necessary in a patient that suffers from significant iliac artery disease that affects the right and left iliac arteries.

Implanted Ventricular Assist Device

If an individual has been diagnosed with heart failure, he or she may be treated with a mechanism known as a ventricular assist device. If a patient has had a ventricular assist device implanted, the vascular technologist can expect to see flow patterns that are modified from what is typically seen. The flow patterns can differ based on which ventricular assist device is used. The most common apparatus used is the left ventricular assist device, which results in a nonpulsatile spectral waveform because continuous flow pumps are used. The PSV and EDV will not be measured due to the nonpulsatility. One end of the device is affixed to the left ventricle with the other end attached to the aorta. If the patient has a biventricular assist device, the spectral analysis will depend on if the flow pump is continuous or pulsatile, which can severely underestimate PSVs.

Transplanted Organs

Liver Transplants

Postoperative Complications

When evaluating a patient that is status post liver transplant, there are several complications that the vascular technologist should evaluate for. It is especially concerning when liver function tests are abnormal postoperatively, and the vascular technologist will be evaluating the liver vasculature for signs of thrombosis, stenosis, or the development of pseudoaneurysms. This evaluation is completed with gray-scale, color, and pulsed-wave Doppler evaluation of the major vessels of the liver and those that supply and drain the digestive system. It is also necessary to evaluate the IVC. If the patient is having pain, nausea, vomiting, or has a fever, it is important to check for perihepatic fluid collections, which may indicate seromas or hematomas, abscesses, or narrowing and/or dilation of the bile ducts.

Evaluating Patients

A follow-up ultrasound will typically be ordered within the first 24 hours after a patient has undergone surgery for a liver transplant because early awareness of complications may decrease the likelihood of transplant failure. The basic protocol is to evaluate the entire abdomen to check for any fluid collections and any signs of pancreatitis. The liver is evaluated with gray-scale, color, and spectral Doppler. Gray-scale imaging is important for determining the size, echogenicity, and texture of the liver. Gray-scale imaging can also be used to initially check the vessels of the liver as well and measure the diameter of the portal vein and to check for any dilation of the bile ducts. Color and spectral Doppler provide important information regarding patency and the direction of blood flow and to evaluate for any turbulence within the main portal vein and its intrahepatic branches, the hepatic veins, and the main hepatic artery as well as its intrahepatic arterial branches and the IVC. It is important to evaluate the anastomoses as well. The PSV, resistive index (RI), and acceleration time measurements should be calculated during spectral Doppler interrogation with special attention given to angle correction.

Copyright © Mometrix Media. You have been licensed one copy of this document for personal use only. Any other reproduction or redistribution is strictly prohibited. All rights reserved.
This content is provided for test preparation purposes only and does not imply an endorsement by Mometrix of any particular political, scientific, or religious point of view.

Renal Transplants

Preferred Location

Most renal transplants are implanted in the iliac fossa of the recipient, with the right iliac fossa being the preferred location. Typically, the left kidney of the donor is removed because the length of the left renal vein is longer than the right. The left kidney is then rotated and implanted into the right iliac fossa. This region is used because it does not interfere with any of the abdominal or pelvic organs, and it is in close proximity to the urinary bladder, which will allow a shorter segment of the ureter to be used and still be inserted above the point at which the native ureter enters the urinary bladder. The iliac fossa is also close to the blood vessels of the iliac region such as the external iliac vein and the internal iliac artery as the transplanted artery needs. Also, this location does not require the removal of the native kidney, which means less risk of infection.

Postoperative Evaluation

It is important for the vascular technologist to look at the patient's medical records in order to determine the approach that should be used for the anastomosis used during his or her renal transplant, and, when available, comparisons should always be made to any prior exams. If the surgery is performed as a live-donor renal transplant, typically the graft of the renal artery will be connected end to end with the internal iliac artery or an end-to-side anastomosis will be formed with the external iliac artery. When the kidney is harvested from a cadaver, the main renal artery is removed with part of the aorta to create an end-to-side connection to the external iliac artery of the recipient. An end-to-side anastomosis approach is the most frequently used connection of the renal vein to the external iliac vein. The ureter of the donor usually enters the dome of the urinary bladder, although sometimes it may be necessary to use the ureter of the recipient. Notably, if the cadaver donor is younger than five years old, both of the kidneys may be implanted into the same recipient.

Diagnosing Rejection

Many physicians rely on a renal biopsy to diagnose rejection of the transplanted kidney. However, when a sonogram is ordered to evaluate for rejection of the transplant, the vascular technologist should use gray-scale ultrasound to measure the maximum size of the kidney in the longitudinal and transverse planes. Any fluid collections should also be documented if present. It is important to compare the results of this study with any previous ultrasounds that have been performed to determine if there is an increase in size. The echogenicity of the cortex of the transplanted kidney should also be evaluated to determine if it is more echogenic, which is also an indication of rejection. The transplanted kidney should also be evaluated for signs of hydronephrosis, and documentation of the level of obstruction should be determined, if possible. Duplex scanning can be used to provide information about complications such as thrombosis of the renal vein, stenosis of the renal artery, and if an AVF has occurred. Some labs will measure the resistivity index to determine an acute rejection, but this is not widely accepted.

Copyright © Mometrix Media. You have been licensed one copy of this document for personal use only. Any other reproduction or redistribution is strictly prohibited. All rights reserved.
This content is provided for test preparation purposes only and does not imply an endorsement by Mometrix of any particular political, scientific, or religious point of view.

Non-Removal of Kidneys

Kidney transplants do not typically require the removal of the patient's native kidneys. If the kidneys do not need to be removed, this may mean an easier recovery for the patient. It can take up to eight weeks for a patient to recover when the native kidneys must be taken out, and more incisions increase the risk of infection. Another concern of removing the native kidneys is the necessity of a blood transfusion because this may prompt antibodies to form, which could be a detriment to the transplanted kidney, but these concerns are decreased if the native kidneys need to be removed after the transplant. The native kidneys are not usually removed unless the patient has cancer or polycystic kidneys, which creates an enlargement of the kidneys due to the multiple cysts.

Copyright © Mometrix Media. You have been licensed one copy of this document for personal use only. Any other reproduction or redistribution is strictly prohibited. All rights reserved.
This content is provided for test preparation purposes only and does not imply an endorsement by Mometrix of any particular political, scientific, or religious point of view.

Physiologic Examinations

Arterial Examinations

Manually Calculate Pressure Indices

Nonimaging Physiologic Exam vs. Duplex Ultrasound Study

A nonimaging physiologic exam is performed to test at least one region of the extremities to determine the presence of disease as well as the significance. Physiologic exams are considered to be indirect studies, but the vascular technologist should always examine the right and left sides so comparisons can be made. Physiologic exams should include the ankle-brachial indices (ABIs) to be calculated by obtaining continuous-wave or pulse volume recordings at the wrist or ankle level. Duplex ultrasound studies involve the use of color and spectral Doppler interrogation and allow for direct evaluation of disease within a specific section of the artery. Duplex ultrasound studies should also be performed bilaterally in order to offer a comparison for a more detailed diagnosis.

Segmental Doppler Pressure

Physicians will order a segmental Doppler pressure as a screening exam to evaluate issues that the patient has with circulation. Segmental pressures are commonly ordered because they are a noninvasive exam to assess the blood flow within the arteries of the extremities. This test can help determine if PAD is present, and in patients that have known PAD, the advancement of the disease can be tracked and compared with prior studies. Segmental Doppler pressures can also help determine if an artery is diseased (and can provide clues to the approximate location), and they can also be used to determine any surgical treatments that may be necessary such as bypass grafting. As a screening exam, segmental pressures will provide clues as to whether an artery is stenosed or occluded (although it cannot discern between the two).

Importance of Rest Prior to Exam

When performing physiologic arterial exams, it may be taxing for the patient to make his or her way back to the ultrasound lab, so it is important to have the patient rest before starting the exam. By allowing the patient to rest for at least five minutes (even more time is better) before the vascular technologist starts the exam, this should provide sufficient time for the blood flow to return to normal before the start of the exam. If this rest time is not afforded to the patient, incorrect testing results could be made. While the vascular technologist is explaining the exam to the patient, the patient should be instructed to lie on his or her back and place the arms down by their sides. The head of the bed can be raised slightly in order to allow the patient to rest comfortably. It is important to be aware of the temperature of the room as well as keeping the patient covered if he or she is cold.

Copyright © Mometrix Media. You have been licensed one copy of this document for personal use only. Any other reproduction or redistribution is strictly prohibited. All rights reserved.
This content is provided for test preparation purposes only and does not imply an endorsement by Mometrix of any particular political, scientific, or religious point of view.

Ankle-Brachial Index

An ankle-brachial index (ABI) is often one of the first tests performed to help screen for PAD when clinically indicated and the findings can help physicians determine if it is mild or severe. These indices are calculated to determine if there is a drop of pressure distal to an artery that is significantly stenosed and is a ratio that compares the blood pressure findings of the lower extremities to the body's overall blood pressure (also referred to as the systemic blood pressure). For ABI calculations, various systolic pressures are recorded in multiple arteries of the lower extremities and the highest arterial pressure on one side of the ankle will be divided by the highest arterial pressure from the highest measurement of the brachial artery. Although it doesn't tell clinicians exactly where the stenosis or occlusion is, it can help narrow down the location.

In order to calculate the ABI, the vascular technologist will first obtain bilateral brachial pressures of the arms. The pressure reading that is the highest will be used later to calculate the ABI value. Two pressures within the ankle are also taken, and the highest reading will be used to calculate the ABI. The two arteries that are used in the ankle region are the DPA and the PTA. Once the pressures are obtained on each side, the vascular technologist may calculate the ABI by taking the highest pressure reading of either the DPA or PTA and dividing it by the highest brachial pressure of either the right or left arm.

Peripheral Resistance and the Pulse Amplitude

An arterial pressure wave is the typical type of energy that is created when blood is flowing in the human body. As blood is pumped out of the heart, the arteries become distended, but the arterioles do not respond with the same amount of distension. Because of the lack of elastin in the arterioles, in diastole the pressure energy is converted to kinetic energy. When vasoconstriction takes place, the peripheral resistance increases distally and a greater amount of the pressure energy in the proximal portion of the arterial vessels will be reflected. This equates to an increase of the pulse amplitude of the arterial wave when it is added to the energy that is already present in the arteries that are in a more proximal location.

Hyperemia with and Without Arterial Obstruction

Hyperemia refers to an increased amount of blood flow to a limb (or any part of the body). If a patient experiences hyperemia in the presence of arterial obstruction, this condition tends to extend the amount of time that this occurs. In patients without a significant arterial obstruction, the hyperemia would take less time for the patient to recover after exercise. If the patient is unable to walk on the treadmill due to conditions such as breathing issues, heart problems, needs the assistance of a walker, or cannot walk for enough time to reproduce the symptoms that he or she has been having, then the reactive hyperemia technique may be used. This method should not be used, however, if the patient has a stent or a bypass graft because it requires the inflation of thigh cuffs to high levels creating too much pressure on the thigh.

Copyright © Mometrix Media. You have been licensed one copy of this document for personal use only. Any other reproduction or redistribution is strictly prohibited. All rights reserved.
This content is provided for test preparation purposes only and does not imply an endorsement by Mometrix of any particular political, scientific, or religious point of view.

Various Sounds Present in Arteries and Veins

Vascular technologists will typically be able to discern the various sounds that are present in arteries and veins. An arterial Doppler of the upper and lower extremities will show a pulsatile, high-frequency signal. A significant stenosis may be heard as an even higher pitched sound than a normal artery because the blood that is moving through the constricted lumen has increased velocities. Vascular technologists will also be able to tell when the transducer is placed in a more proximal and distal location to the segment of the artery that is stenotic. Recall that audible venous sounds will change with respiration and are usually considered to be of low frequency.

Obtaining Appropriate Diagnostic Waveforms/Pressures

Required Exercise During the Exam

When a patient describes symptoms of claudication, but the segmental pressure exam is within normal limits (or when the results are borderline normal), then protocols typically involve having the patient exercise whenever possible. Another reason that patients are required to exercise is if they have already been diagnosed with arterial disease but the extent of the disease during exercise has not yet been determined. The vascular technologist will typically calculate ABIs first without exercise. Immediately after the patient stops exercising, ABIs are calculated every two minutes until the results are restored to the numbers calculated before the patient walked on the treadmill. If the patient is unable to walk on the treadmill, it is possible to have them perform toe raises during the exercise phase.

Claudication and Cardiac Treadmill Exercise Exams

Regardless of the type of exercise exams performed, it is important for the sonographer to closely monitor the patient and his or her blood pressure. When the patient is required to exercise for symptoms of claudication, he or she will be asked to walk on a treadmill until the pain becomes unbearable or for no more than five minutes. The treadmill is usually set with an incline of 12%, and the speed will be between 1.5 and 2 mph (2 mph is preferred), but once the speed is set it does not typically change. The goal of cardiac treadmill exercise testing is to achieve a target heart rate that is determined for this patient, which can be achieved by increasing the incline and speed of the treadmill during various times throughout the study.

Time of Recovery and Diagnosis

If the patient is asked to exercise, the vascular technologist has already performed pre-exercise testing ABIs and pressure readings. Post-exercise testing ABIs and pressures are attained right after the patient is done exercising and then at two-minute intervals until the pre-exercise values are reached. Determination of a single level or more than one level can be discerned by comparing the pre- and postexercise values. If the patient's pressures reach the pre-exercise numbers in less than 5 minutes, this suggests that the patient only has disease in one level. Disease in more than one level is suggested when it takes more than 12 minutes for the pre-exercise levels to be reached. Normal post-exercise findings include an increase of the ABIs and the pressure values. If the pressure readings fall below those that were

Copyright © Mometrix Media. You have been licensed one copy of this document for personal use only. Any other reproduction or redistribution is strictly prohibited. All rights reserved.
This content is provided for test preparation purposes only and does not imply an endorsement by Mometrix of any particular political, scientific, or religious point of view.

obtained while the patient was at rest, it suggests that disease is present, with more significant disease equating to a greater decline in pressure readings.

Effect of Making a Fist

If a patient is asked to make a fist during an upper extremity Doppler exam, the waveform of the brachial artery will likely appear more pulsatile, which, in turn, results in a higher pulsatility index. Recall that the pulsatility index offers quantitative information and can be calculated by the following formula: $\frac{\text{PS}-\text{ED}}{\text{mean}}$, where PS is the peak-systolic velocity, ED is the end-diastolic velocity, and mean represents the mean velocity. Typically, less distal resistance will demonstrate a waveform with low pulsatility, and high resistance will demonstrate a waveform that has increased pulsatility. Having the patient make a fist will create more resistance in the arteries that are found in a more distal location of the upper extremity, and the vascular technologist will also notice that the amount of diastolic blood flow has likely been reduced.

Select the Appropriate Instrumentation

Inflating the Blood Pressure Cuff

During Doppler pressure exams, the vascular technologist should start by taking bilateral brachial arterial pressures and documenting both readings. The vascular technologist must remember the highest brachial pressure reading because this value will be used not only to calculate the ABIs, but also when taking other pressure measurements. For example, the cuff should be inflated 20–30 mmHg more than the highest brachial arterial systolic pressure. Once the arterial Doppler sound is no longer heard, the vascular technologist should continue to increase the blood pressure cuff pressure 20–30 mmHg higher than this point. If it is determined that the pressures must be repeated, the sonographer should wait for roughly a minute after deflation of the cuff to allow the blood flow to return to the artery because if the next pressure reading is taken too soon, it could be miscalculated at a value lower than the actual reading.

Vascular technologists must consider the size of blood pressure cuffs that are chosen for each patient and the area of the extremities used for pressure readings. Vascular labs will typically have their chosen protocols regarding the number of cuffs that are used (either the three- or four-cuff methods). When performing pressure measurements of the upper extremities, there will typically be three cuffs that are applied to the wrist, forearm, and upper arm. The wrist cuff used is usually 5–10 cm, the forearm cuff chosen will usually be a 10 cm cuff, with a 12 cm cuff being selected for the upper arm. Exams of the lower extremities may either be three- or four-cuff techniques with the ankle and calf level using a 10 cm cuff, if a three-cuff method is used, a 17–19 cm cuff is applied to the thigh, and if a four-cuff method is chosen, then the sonographer should select a 12 cm for the upper and lower region of the thigh.

Copyright © Mometrix Media. You have been licensed one copy of this document for personal use only. Any other reproduction or redistribution is strictly prohibited. All rights reserved.
This content is provided for test preparation purposes only and does not imply an endorsement by Mometrix of any particular political, scientific, or religious point of view.

Calculating the ABI in the Calf

To determine the ABI, the vascular technologist will record the pressures at the ankle level of the PTA as well as the DPA. An ABI is calculated separately for the PTA and DPA by dividing these pressures by the highest brachial arterial pressure that was recorded from both arms. However, the highest calculated ABI will be calculated and used for each side. An ABI will be calculated bilaterally for comparison. Notably, ankle pressures are typically equal to or greater than the blood pressure reading of the brachial artery that is the highest. When performing lower extremity exams, the pressure measurements should be performed in the distal leg first and then moved proximally.

Obtaining Segmental Pressures

When a patient is having a segmental pressure exam, it is important to have the patient lie on the ultrasound table in a supine position. A pillow should be offered to the patient (and the head of the bed can be raised just slightly if the patient is uncomfortable with just a pillow), but the goal is to have the heart and extremities in the same plane. The patient should be instructed to relax the legs so they are straight, and the arms should be down by the sides. The reason that the heart and extremities should be in roughly the same plane with the patient supine is to overcome the response to hydrostatic pressure because the pressure of the ankle increases when the patient stands because it depends on the distance of the artery from the heart as well as the force of gravity. As long as the patient is supine, there is only a slight effect of hydrostatic pressure witnessed within the arteries and veins.

Cuff Artifacts

While performing segmental pressures, sonographers must take extra care in choosing the size of the cuff for each patient and the size of their extremities in order to avoid cuff artifact. A cuff artifact can lead to a misdiagnosis of the patient because it can mistakenly create pressures that are either too high or too low. The width of the cuff should be at least 20% greater than the patient's extremity. If the cuff is not wide enough, for example, during a lower extremity exam, it could result in a pressure reading that is higher than it should be. If the cuff is too large, then a low-pressure reading will likely occur. If a four-cuff method is used, it is important to note that if a cuff artifact is present it is usually found in the high thigh with the pressure being 30 mmHg greater than the brachial arterial pressure that was found to be a higher value.

Photoplethysmography

Photoplethysmography (PPG) is often used to determine if arterial disease is present in the digits (fingers and toes) by sending an infrared light into the prominent tissue of the finger so the light that is reflected will represent the amount of cutaneous blood flow. Prior to the exam, it is important that the vascular technologist determine if the patient is anxious about the exam because the results can be skewed if this is the case because stress can induce a narrowing of the arteries and affect blood pressure. Answering all questions that the patient may have about the test so he or she knows what to expect should alleviate the amount

Copyright © Mometrix Media. You have been licensed one copy of this document for personal use only. Any other reproduction or redistribution is strictly prohibited. All rights reserved.
This content is provided for test preparation purposes only and does not imply an endorsement by Mometrix of any particular political, scientific, or religious point of view.

of nervousness that is felt. It is important that the vascular technologist also asks if the patient is cold because vasoconstriction will alter the effectiveness of the test. Yet another factor that impacts the arteries to cause vasoconstriction is smoking, so it is important to find out if the patient has smoked recently.

Evaluating Fingers with Plethysmography

If a physician is trying to rule out Raynaud's phenomenon, the vascular technologist may need to examine the patient's fingers with and without cold stress. The technique first evaluates the patient without cold stress while keeping the patient warm. In order to eliminate the possibility of disease in the proximal vessels, the sonographer should obtain bilateral brachial artery pressures as well as pressures of the forearm. Recall that the ulnar and radial arteries deliver oxygenated blood to the hand, so it is necessary to also evaluate the palmar arch. The fingertips of the digits that are of concern will be evaluated by waveform and pressure plethysmography. For the cold stress, the patient's hands will be placed in ice water until it becomes unbearable or for a maximum of three minutes. It is important to note any changes in skin color or symptoms that the patient has as well as how long the patient's hands were immersed in the ice water. Although the exam is performed bilaterally, if one side is of greater concern, that side should be examined first. The same method is used immediately after wiping off the water and is repeated again five minutes later.

Using Cold Stress

Cold stress PPG testing is an important method to perform if true vasospasm is suspected in an individual because the blood flow to the digits can be normal when the patient is tested without cold stress. With this evaluation, the waveforms and pressures should be performed at room temperature with the patient at a comfortable temperature. Cold stress testing requires the patient to place their hands in ice water for three minutes or until it becomes unbearable. It is considered abnormal if the patient's waveforms do not return to the levels of those that were seen before cold stress was applied by the five-minute mark. Normally, the amplitude of the waveform is hardly impacted by the ice water, but when the patient experiences vasospasm, the peaks demonstrate a rounded appearance.

Obtaining Toe Pressures

The method used to obtain toe pressures is usually done in conjunction with a physiologic arterial exam of the lower extremities. However, if ordered separately, it is important to eliminate the possibility of disease in the proximal arteries, so bilateral ABIs will be calculated first. Either volume or photoplethysmographic waveforms are obtained from the great toes as well as any other toes that are of concern. Some labs use continuous-wave Doppler for the pressures with volume or photo techniques, but this can be technically challenging because it can be difficult to stay on the tiny digital arteries. The cuff will be placed at the base of the great toe, and the photocell is applied to the undersurface of the distal portion of the same digit. The sonographer will inflate the cuff at the same time that the arterial pulses are being recorded. Once the cuff is 20–30 mmHg more than the highest ankle

Copyright © Mometrix Media. You have been licensed one copy of this document for personal use only. Any other reproduction or redistribution is strictly prohibited. All rights reserved.
This content is provided for test preparation purposes only and does not imply an endorsement by Mometrix of any particular political, scientific, or religious point of view.

pressure systolic reading, the pulsation should stop, which prompts the technologist to deflate the cuff. When the pulse appears again in the PPG tracing, the toe pressure is documented.

Normal Limits of Fingers and Toes

Normal PPG studies that are performed of the fingers and toes are considered to be within normal limits if the waveform demonstrates a sharp upstroke at the same time of peak systole. There should also be a downstroke that is lengthy with a dicrotic notch visualized about halfway through the downstroke. It is important to note that the waveforms of the toes tend to have a smaller amplitude when compared to the amplitude of the fingers. Abnormal qualities include a slow upstroke, with a dicrotic notch appearing in a high location of the downstroke (instead of halfway down). If an occlusion is present proximally to the most distal portion of the digit, the waveform will tend to have a more rounded appearance of the peak with a slow upstroke. Raynaud's phenomenon often demonstrates a PPG waveform that has a peaked pulse.

Copyright © Mometrix Media. You have been licensed one copy of this document for personal use only. Any other reproduction or redistribution is strictly prohibited. All rights reserved.
This content is provided for test preparation purposes only and does not imply an endorsement by Mometrix of any particular political, scientific, or religious point of view.

Venous Examinations

Obtaining Appropriate Venous PPG Diagnostic Waveforms

Advantages and Disadvantages of PPG

PPG uses a photocell that is placed slightly above the medial malleolus while the patient is sitting with his or her legs hanging off the table. This modality is a noninvasive test that can be used to evaluate venous and arterial blood flow. The venous PPG will use the DC mode because it detects blood that is moving more slowly. PPG is used to determine if venous insufficiency is present and its significance. The photocell should not be used in areas of skin that are broken or ulcerated, and it should not be placed over a varicose vein because doing so can provide false data. Another problem that the vascular technologist may encounter is that unusually thick skin may hinder the propagation of the infrared light into the subcutaneous tissue.

Dorsiflexion Maneuver During

While the patient sits upright with his or her legs hanging off the table, the vascular technologist will ask the patient to dorsiflex the foot. During these studies with various maneuvers, the vascular technologist may have to demonstrate the action for the patient or give very specific instructions. The patient should perform an exaggerated dorsiflexion 5 to 10 times so the blood empties from the veins. In some cases, the individual may not be able to dorsiflex the foot well enough, so the sonographer can squeeze the calf for them. If manual compression is necessary on one side, the vascular technologist must perform this for the patent bilaterally in order to obtain comparable results. The venous refill time is obtained after completing the dorsiflexion exercises.

Air Plethysmography

Air plethysmography is also referred to as volume plethysmography. This modality can be used for venous and arterial testing. Venous applications are used to determine if CVI is present by determining the venous filling index, the ejection fraction, and the residual volume fraction while evaluating the patient in various positions and movements. This study is important to determine the filling of the veins as well as the depletion of the venous blood. The exam is performed after the application of a cuff that encircles the calf region first with the patient supine. The patient is then instructed to stand quickly for a couple of more measurements/movements and then will return to the supine position to deplete the blood from the veins once again.

Venous Filling Index

During an air plethysmography exam, once the vascular technologist determines the zero venous volume, the sonographer will ask the patient to stand up quickly from the supine position. The patient's test leg should be non-weight-bearing. Gravity will enable the blood to fill the veins of the lower leg once again. Then, the venous filling

Copyright © Mometrix Media. You have been licensed one copy of this document for personal use only. Any other reproduction or redistribution is strictly prohibited. All rights reserved.
This content is provided for test preparation purposes only and does not imply an endorsement by Mometrix of any particular political, scientific, or religious point of view.

index (VFI) can be calculated to determine how fast the veins refill. The VFI is calculated using the following formula:

$$\text{VFI} = \frac{90\%\ \text{venous volume}}{90\%\ \text{venous filling time}}.$$

A VFI of less than or equal to 2 is considered normal. If the VFI falls in the 2–10 range, it suggests that a minor to moderate reflux is present. If the VFI is greater than 10, then it is assumed that the patient has severe reflux.

NORMAL EJECTION FRACTION

When performing an air plethysmography study, it is considered normal if the ejection fraction (EF) is greater than 60%. After the venous filling index is found after the patient quickly stands from the supine position, the patient will stand on both feet and will be asked to exercise in order to stimulate the calf-muscle pump. This can be performed by asking the patient to perform one calf raise by having the patient stand on their tiptoes to the best of their ability. The EF is calculated with the following formula:

$$\text{EF} = \frac{\text{EV}}{\text{VV}} \times 100,$$

where EV is the ejection volume and VV is the venous volume.

RESIDUAL VOLUME FRACTION

When performing an air plethysmography study, the residual volume fraction (RVF) is one of the parameters that is calculated. A study is considered to be normal when the RVF is calculated to be less than 35%. The RVF is calculated after the EF (in which the patient performs 1 calf raise), and the vascular technologist will ask the patient to perform 10 more calf raises. This value determines how much blood remains in the veins after having the patient perform this maneuver. The RVF is the ratio of the residual volume to the venous volume:

$$\text{RVF} = \frac{\text{RV}}{\text{VV}}.$$

KNOWLEDGE AND SKILLS

VENOUS REFILL TIME

If the results of the venous refill time (VRT) is greater than or equal to 20 seconds, then the PPG study is determined to be within normal limits. If the VRT is less than 20 seconds, the exam is considered abnormal. If this is the case, the sonographer would continue the exam by wrapping a tourniquet around the patient's distal thigh region and the patient is instructed to dorsiflex his or her foot 5 to 10 times. The VRT is obtained once again, and if it is greater than 20 seconds then it is assumed that reflux is present in the GSV. The sonographer should continue the exam by applying the tourniquet just below the knee and asking the patient to dorsiflex the foot 5 to 10 times and repeat the tracings. At this point, it can be discerned that if the VRT is greater than 20 seconds with the tourniquet in place inferior to the knee

Copyright © Mometrix Media. You have been licensed one copy of this document for personal use only. Any other reproduction or redistribution is strictly prohibited. All rights reserved.
This content is provided for test preparation purposes only and does not imply an endorsement by Mometrix of any particular political, scientific, or religious point of view.

that reflux is present in the SSV. It is suggested that incompetence of the deep system is present when a VRT of less than 20 seconds is found with and without the use of the tourniquet.

Copyright © Mometrix Media. You have been licensed one copy of this document for personal use only. Any other reproduction or redistribution is strictly prohibited. All rights reserved.
This content is provided for test preparation purposes only and does not imply an endorsement by Mometrix of any particular political, scientific, or religious point of view.

Ultrasound-Guided Procedures/ Intraoperative Assessment

Participate in Manual Compression of Pseudoaneurysms

More radiographic procedures are being performed, which translates to more pseudoaneurysm formation, especially of the CFA. Ultrasound can be used to diagnose this condition, but it can also be used as a guide during compression. The size of the aneurysm should be documented along with the diameter of the neck. Gray-scale and color Doppler should be used to make sure that the transducer is compressing the neck so blood cannot move into the sac while still enabling the blood to flow into the femoral artery. This compression should take roughly 10 to 20 minutes, and it can be applied with the ultrasound transducer. After this time frame, the pressure can be released to see if there has been clotting of the pseudoaneurysm.

Provide Guidance for Thrombin Injections of Pseudoaneurysms

Ultrasound is not only a great modality to diagnose a pseudoaneurysm, but it is also a great tool to help monitor this pulsatile mass to determine if it will clot on its own. Sometimes surgical repair is necessary for pseudoaneurysms, but most of the time compression or percutaneous thrombin injections are useful, with thrombin injection being the most common procedure that is done. Gray-scale and color Doppler ultrasound are used during the injection process until it appears as if the pseudoaneurysm is clotted. Once there is an absence of flow when monitoring with color Doppler, it is assumed that thrombosis has taken place. The vascular technologist should also document images of the proximal and distal arteries of this pulsatile mass.

Provide Guidance for Venous Ablation Procedures

Ultrasound Prior to Ablation

The role that ultrasound plays prior to an ablation is to diagnose which sections of the varicose veins demonstrate reflux. The depth of the vessels should also be noted to determine any necessary precautions that may need to be taken to prevent extensive tissue damage. The size of the vessel must be measured to help determine if ablation can take place. Vascular technologists can map how the vein travels as well as document how far this blood vessel is from the GSV. Documentation should also include the distance from the vein of interest distally to the region of the knee.

Ultrasound During Ablation

The vascular technologist will assist during an ablation procedure by setting up the tray and collecting the necessary supplies. The patient should be placed on the table and prepped, and sterile drapes should be used. The role of ultrasound for guidance should be to image the site that will be used. Often, if the access site is the GSV, then just above or below the knee is where the catheter or laser fiber will be placed. The ankle or distal calf region will be the area of placement if the SSV is of interest.

Copyright © Mometrix Media. You have been licensed one copy of this document for personal use only. Any other reproduction or redistribution is strictly prohibited. All rights reserved.
This content is provided for test preparation purposes only and does not imply an endorsement by Mometrix of any particular political, scientific, or religious point of view.

Ultrasound should be used to make sure that the tool is 2–3 cm from the saphenofemoral location. Care should be taken so the catheter is not in the femoral vein because this could create a DVT if the vein is damaged. Anesthesia should be given, and ultrasound can document the correct placement so the patient will not feel as much heat and to prevent burns of the skin. Once the procedure is over, the catheter or laser fiber is taken out.

Obtain Appropriate Postprocedural Diagnostic Images

Indications for a Postoperative Hemodialysis Access

Due to the high failure rate postoperatively within the first year for postoperative hemodialysis access, ultrasound imaging may be necessary to aid clinicians to determine if the access site is functioning even when the clinical exam appears normal. Common indications for an ultrasound evaluation of the hemodialysis access site is if a blood flow rate of 400 mL/min cannot be achieved or if bleeding occurs longer than expected post dialysis even when pressure is applied. Another indication for imaging is if the AVF does not mature even after at least six weeks. An ultrasound will be ordered postoperatively if the patient has pain or swelling or has a cold hand or fingers after having dialysis or after the surgery has taken place. If a thrill cannot be felt over a fistula or if it appears to be smaller than expected, then an ultrasound evaluation should be performed.

Sites for an AVF in the Upper Extremity

The radial artery and cephalic vein are common sites for an arteriovenous fistula (AVF) in the upper extremity because the forearm is favored over the use of the upper arm whenever possible. Typically, the nondominant forearm is used, and if it fails the dominant forearm is still the preferred access site over the upper arm, but in either case the cephalic vein will serve as the draining vein and will become distended for hemodialysis access. In contrast to an anastomosis created in the upper arm, when a hemodialysis access of the forearm is used, it is in a more superficial location than those of the upper arm, and this typically equates to less discomfort for the patient because it is easier to cannulate when the patient undergoes dialysis. Also, if the forearm access sites become thrombosed and fail, it is still possible to create a new access site more proximally, whereas the reverse situation does not typically work. If an access site in the upper arm is created first and fails, it is not likely that a forearm or more distal access site will be able to be used on the same arm.

Stenosis Is Suspected in an Upper Extremity AVF

If stenosis of an upper extremity AVF is suspected, the vascular technologist has several steps to complete because the fistula along with the anastomosis, draining vein, arterial inflow, as well as evaluate for any fluid collections should be done. The diameter of the fistula should be the first thing that is documented, and this can be evaluated with gray-scale ultrasound. The PSV ratio of the anastomosis/artery 2 cm upstream should be calculated as well. The draining vein should be assessed with gray-scale, color, and spectral Doppler. Stenosis or even thrombosis is suspected of the cranial system if there is little to no flow in the draining vein. Once again, the

Copyright © Mometrix Media. You have been licensed one copy of this document for personal use only. Any other reproduction or redistribution is strictly prohibited. All rights reserved.
This content is provided for test preparation purposes only and does not imply an endorsement by Mometrix of any particular political, scientific, or religious point of view.

PSV ratio is calculated, but this time it is the comparison of the narrowed draining vein to the vein 2 cm upstream. The subclavian and internal jugular veins should be examined with spectral Doppler to check for stenosis as well. Although stenosis of the inflow artery is fairly unusual, the feeding artery should also be evaluated.

AVF That Has Failed to Mature

When scanning a patient postoperatively because their AVF has not matured even after four to eight weeks post surgery, the goal is to determine if there is an anatomic issue that can be repaired. The anastomosis is scanned to determine if it is stenotic. The draining vein should be evaluated with gray-scale, color, and spectral Doppler as well to see if a stenosis is present. The diameter of the AVF should be measured and should be at least 4 mm in order for it to be functional. Volume blood flow measurements are taken as well in the straightest segment possible that does not show turbulence and is in the middle of the draining vein. Calculations of 500–600 mL/min tend to have a high affinity for a positive outcome for this AVF to use for hemodialysis.

Copyright © Mometrix Media. You have been licensed one copy of this document for personal use only. Any other reproduction or redistribution is strictly prohibited. All rights reserved.
This content is provided for test preparation purposes only and does not imply an endorsement by Mometrix of any particular political, scientific, or religious point of view.

Quality Assurance, Safety, and Physical Principles

Quality Assurance and Safety

Assess the Appropriateness of the Exam

Implementing a QA Program Vascular Labs

Vascular ultrasound labs must immediately incorporate a quality improvement program that includes quality assurance (QA) as one of the components. This is an ongoing program that is put into place to make sure that patient outcomes coincide with the results that are reported from the procedures taking place. The QA program also allows policies and protocols to be put into place. The protocols should identify which vessels each vascular technologist is expected to examine and how abnormalities should be documented. Other examples of what a QA program can do is to decrease the number of times a patient must return for additional studies, minimize exams that are not of superior diagnostic quality, and to ensure that scanning criteria are being met by every vascular technologist and interpreting physician. This documentation must be available in cases of lawsuits to prove that the images and measurement tools are satisfactory.

Reviewing Physician's Written or Electronic Order

Prior to completing an ultrasound exam, the sonographer should carefully review the written (or electronic) order to determine why a particular exam is being requested. The ordering physician should clearly state the indications for the exam that is requested. If the vascular technologist does not think that the correct exam has been ordered after discussing symptoms with the patient, it can be addressed with the radiologist (or the interpreting physician) who can contact the ordering physician to determine if a different test may be more appropriate. The written or electronic order must include the name and date of birth of the patient, the exam that is being ordered, as well as the indications for the procedure. The order must also include the signature of the physician as well as a phone number, fax number, and address so the written report is sent to the correct provider.

Reasons for Another Carotid Duplex to Be Ordered

In most cases, it is believed to be unnecessary to perform another carotid duplex exam on the same patient unless that individual has experienced additional symptoms in which the physician wants to have the carotid duplex exam repeated in order to better treat the patient. Some of the things that a patient may report as worsening symptoms and affect the anterior circulation are problems speaking and amaurosis fugax. Symptoms that affect the posterior circulation include double vision and dysphagia with or without vertigo. If it has been established that a patient has experienced moderate (50%–69%) stenosis, they should undergo a

Copyright © Mometrix Media. You have been licensed one copy of this document for personal use only. Any other reproduction or redistribution is strictly prohibited. All rights reserved.
This content is provided for test preparation purposes only and does not imply an endorsement by Mometrix of any particular political, scientific, or religious point of view.

follow-up study every year. For those that have severe (70%–99%) stenosis, it is recommended that a follow-up ultrasound should be performed every six months.

Following the ALARA Principle

Vascular technologists must always keep the as low as reasonably achievable (ALARA) principle in mind when performing exams. Many people associate this concept with radiation, but it is also an important assumption for all ultrasound users as well. For example, if an entire image is too bright, the most effective way to decrease patient exposure is to decrease the output power (also known as the acoustic power). When there is a reduction in the power setting, there is a decrease in the voltage applied to the ultrasound transducer, which, in turn, decreases the amount of energy that the patient is exposed to. The vascular technologist could also turn down the overall gain to prevent an image from being too bright, but it is important to understand that gain has no effect on patient exposure. However, if an image is too dark, the best choice for adhering to the ALARA principle is to increase the gain because it does not affect the energy imparted to the patient.

Greatest Impact on Patient Exposure

Ultrasound should only be used for clinical exams in which the benefits outweigh the risks. One risk during an exam is an elevation of temperature in tissues exposed to the ultrasound beam. One of the parameters that the vascular technologist should watch is the thermal index (TI), and it is understood that it will be highest during an exam with a high-frequency, high-intensity beam. This heating depends on the exposure time and temperature. Typically, the greatest increase in temperature is witnessed with spectral Doppler exams. Pulsed-wave Doppler requires more energy than B-mode or gray-scale imaging. Ideally, the TI should be 1.0 or less and the time should be minimized to prevent tissue heating. If the TI is 1.0, there is a possibility that the temperature of the tissue will increase by 1 degree. TI is expressed by the soft-tissue thermal index (TIS), bone thermal index (TIB), and cranial bone thermal index (TIC).

Decreasing the MI

The mechanical index (MI) reading on an ultrasound machine determines the probability of bioeffects when gas bubbles in the tissue interact with the ultrasound beam. This is a phenomenon known as cavitation. The significance of a system displaying a high MI is that there is a better chance that bioeffects will occur. If a vascular technologist notices that the MI is too high, it is helpful to decrease the output power on the machine in order to reduce the amount of voltage sent to the transducer. The operator should also increase the frequency of the transducer because the frequency and MI have an inverse relationship. These adjustments are effective in reducing the display because lower frequency and pressure are two properties of the beam that tend to raise the MI.

How PRF Contributes to Patient Exposure

Vascular technologists should always be cognizant of the ALARA principle during ultrasound exams. Gray-scale imaging exposes the patient to the least amount of

Copyright © Mometrix Media. You have been licensed one copy of this document for personal use only. Any other reproduction or redistribution is strictly prohibited. All rights reserved.
This content is provided for test preparation purposes only and does not imply an endorsement by Mometrix of any particular political, scientific, or religious point of view.

bioeffects. When color and pulsed Doppler are activated, the acoustic exposure risk becomes higher. Of the choices, the pulse repetition frequency (PRF) would contribute to patient exposure because if it is increased, there is less listening time required as the pulses are being transmitted into the body. This increases the risk of acoustic exposure to the patient. If the vascular technologist notices Doppler signals that have become really "noisy," it is because most modern systems have a built-in safety feature that will automatically reduce the output power if the PRF is too high.

Stable vs. Transient Cavitation

Two types of cavitation exist when force and frequency from an ultrasound beam are applied to tissues. These are known as stable and transient cavitation. The MI reading on the machine alerts the sonographer to the possibility that cavitation will create dangerous bioeffects within the tissue being imaged. A smaller MI number indicates that stable cavitation will occur. Stable cavitation is the increasing, decreasing, and vibration of gas bubbles located within tissues when exposed to variations in pressure of the sound wave. These bubbles tend to acquire much of the energy of the sound wave, but they do not rupture. Transient (normal, inertial) cavitation occurs with higher MI readings. In this situation, the microbubbles tend to rupture, creating increased pressure and temperature measurements.

Monitoring the TI During a Sonogram

Patient safety is a primary concern during an ultrasound. Bioeffects can occur if an increase in tissue temperature occurs as a result of the interactions of tissue with the ultrasound beam. The TI is displayed on the screen for users as an indicator of a possible increase in tissue temperature. Research has shown that an increase in temperature of some tissues by as little as two to four degrees can cause bioeffects. This, of course, depends on the tissue type as well as the amount of time that the tissue is exposed. The TI is directly related to the acoustic output of the machine. There are three types of TIs that serve as the best in vivo indicators of a rise in temperature. These are the TIS, TIB, and TIC.

Application Showing Lowest Levels of Tissue Heating

It is no surprise that the lowest level of tissue heating occurs when the output intensity of the equipment being used is at its lowest numerical value. Generally, gray-scale imaging is the method in which tissue heating will be the lowest. Tissue heating is typically the highest when pulsed Doppler is being used. M-mode and color-flow Doppler tend to fall in the midst of these intensities. One way to determine the numerical values of these intensities is to evaluate the sound wave by using a hydrophone. A hydrophone may be used by engineers to measure the output intensities as well as other characteristics of an ultrasound wave. The hydrophone is actually a transducer that is about the size of a needle, which provides accurate values because of its compact size.

Statement on Mammalian Biological Effects of Ultrasound in Vivo

Vascular technologists should be aware that the term "in vivo" involves observing possible bioeffects that take place inside a living body. The spatial peak temporal

Copyright © Mometrix Media. You have been licensed one copy of this document for personal use only. Any other reproduction or redistribution is strictly prohibited. All rights reserved.
This content is provided for test preparation purposes only and does not imply an endorsement by Mometrix of any particular political, scientific, or religious point of view.

average (SPTA) is the intensity that is referred to in the "Statement on Mammalian Biological Effects of Ultrasound In Vivo." Unfavorable outcomes have been observed in exploratory conditions. Many experiments have been carried out in the lab setting pertaining to the possible bioeffects that ultrasound has on the body. Lab mammals are used to help experts better comprehend the associated risks that ultrasound has on the body. Scientists agree that lower ultrasound frequencies pose no threat to human tissue during in vivo trials. During controlled trials, it has been confirmed that as long as a focused beam's SPTA intensity does not go higher than $1W/cm^2$ and an unfocused beam's SPTA intensity stays below $100\ mW/cm^2$, then bioeffects should not occur.

Greatest Risk of Injury to a Patient

Ultrasound labs must perform routine preventative maintenance on their equipment to make sure that all parameters are within the acceptable standards for ultrasound equipment. It is up to the vascular technologist to make sure that all parts of the equipment are inspected on a regular basis. Sonographers should make sure that the machine is plugged into the correct electrical outlets and that the cords do not present a trip hazard. There are many fundamental pieces of the machine that may be connected to the patient at the same time. The transducer is an integral part of the ultrasound machine, and it is the component that is always directly on or within the patient. This contact would account for the greatest risk of injury to the patient during an exam. Not only could a damaged transducer degrade the quality of an image, but a cracked transducer could impart an electrical shock to the patient.

Exam Findings to Correlative Studies Comparison

Often an ultrasound exam may be performed as a follow-up to a disorder that has already been diagnosed with another imaging modality or prior ultrasound. If a patient has had previous imaging (MRI, CT, ultrasound, etc.) completed, it is important to look at the images and read the report so the vascular technologist knows exactly what is to be interrogated. It is also important that the radiologist has this information because ordering physicians appreciate and expect comparative reports. Ultrasound is useful as a follow-up modality because it does not subject the patient to ionizing radiation like CT and X-ray do. Some labs use technology known as fusion imaging, which allows side-by-side ultrasound imaging with comparative CT or MRI studies that have already been performed. This technique allows more confidence that the lesion visualized on ultrasound is the same lesion shown on a previous study.

Collaborate Regarding Exam Protocols

Documentation Compliance

Every vascular lab has its own protocols regarding how procedures are performed, but all of these protocols should include the proper documentation. Documentation begins as the patient first checks in to the facility for his or her exam, and it continues prior to, during, and after the patient has left the facility. All Health Insurance Portability and Accountability Act of 1996 (HIPAA) and necessary consent forms are signed prior to the procedure. The ultrasound exam must be

Copyright © Mometrix Media. You have been licensed one copy of this document for personal use only. Any other reproduction or redistribution is strictly prohibited. All rights reserved.
This content is provided for test preparation purposes only and does not imply an endorsement by Mometrix of any particular political, scientific, or religious point of view.

saved so the images can be reviewed at a later date, if necessary, and it is considered part of the patient's permanent records. A final report is generated by the reading physician. Every effort should be made to ensure that the final report is sent to the ordering physician in a timely fashion so the patient's team can plan and manage their treatment as needed. It is imperative that all of this is done in a manner that preserves patient confidentiality.

Calculating the Accuracy of Vascular Exams

When a department manager needs to calculate the accuracy of vascular exams that are performed in the department, he or she is trying to determine the percentage of studies that are correctly ruling out as well as revealing disease. This includes diagnosing positive studies for disease if a disease does indeed exist. Not only are the positive studies analyzed for accuracy, but the manager will also be looking for normal exams that were diagnosed as normal when the blood flow dynamics are unremarkable. The accuracy can be calculated by taking the total number of exams that matched the diagnosis of the radiologist or interpreting physician and dividing this number by the total number of exams performed in the department. Accuracy is often calculated as part of the QA statistics that the manager must assess.

Includes Sensitivity and Specificity

Sensitivity is an important part of QA: It refers to the capability of noninvasive exam to identify a disease or disorder when compared to the gold standard method. The sensitivity of vascular exams would indicate the number of noninvasive tests that were correctly diagnosed as being positive studies. The sensitivity can be determined by taking the number of correct positive exams and dividing it by the number of positive studies performed by the exam that is considered to be the gold standard for testing. The specificity is the capability of noninvasive exams to discern that a study is normal when compared to the gold standard method. This is calculated by taking the number of noninvasive results that are true negative and dividing this by the number of every negative result that was diagnosed by the gold standard method.

Calculating Positive and Negative Predictive Values

The positive predictive value is calculated by determining the number of noninvasive studies that are true positives and dividing this number by the total number of noninvasive studies that are positive. This value will give the percentage of noninvasive exams that were diagnosed as positive studies when compared to the gold standard exam. These tests were able to find disease that is indeed present in the patient. The negative predictive value is calculated by taking the number of noninvasive exams that are true negative diagnoses divided by the total number of noninvasive exams that are determined to have negative findings. This determines the percentage of noninvasive exams that did not find the presence of disease as confirmed by the gold standard study.

Copyright © Mometrix Media. You have been licensed one copy of this document for personal use only. Any other reproduction or redistribution is strictly prohibited. All rights reserved.
This content is provided for test preparation purposes only and does not imply an endorsement by Mometrix of any particular political, scientific, or religious point of view.

Monitor Patient Condition

Reducing Anxiety

It is important to show empathy during an ultrasound exam. Often, the patient is nervous about the procedure and results, so it is up to the vascular technologist to help the patient feel more comfortable. After correctly identifying the patient, the sonographer should introduce themselves to the patient. Explain the exam that will be performed, and answer any questions that may arise. An important step prior to the exam is to get a thorough medical history from the patient and find out if any prior exams have been done for comparison. Make sure that the patient is as comfortable as possible, and during the exam check in and ask about how he or she is doing. Once the exam is over, make sure the gel is wiped off and help the patient dress if necessary. It is also important to inform the patient how he or she will receive their results and a time frame in which to expect them. A sonographer should not relay any of the associated findings to the patient because results must come from the ordering physician or radiologist. Patients often appreciate being shown back to the waiting room after the exam is finished.

Dizziness

If the patient experiences dizziness and starts to fall, it is important for the vascular technologist to try to prevent the patient from hitting his or her head on anything while slowly assisting the patient to the floor when standing next to the patient. Falls happen very quickly, and the first reflex of the vascular technologist may be to try to catch the patient, which may end up injuring both parties. Sometimes falls take place when the technologist is not standing beside the patient. In that case, call for help and seek immediate medical treatment for the patient if he or she is injured. Some labs may require the radiologist or cardiologist to examine the patient. Along with head trauma, other concerns especially for elderly patients are a fractured hip (or any other bone). Familiarize yourself with policies when these situations arise, and fill out an incident report with specific details of the fall.

Safety Measures

The priority of the vascular technologist when an individual enters the room is patient safety. Although the lights are typically dimmed during an ultrasound exam, they should be bright when the patient enters and exits the room. The pathway to the exam table should be cleared of any objects to prevent a trip hazard, and, if possible, the patient should have access to the table from the side that is opposite the ultrasound machine. Most labs have adjustable tables that can move up and down; the table should be lowered to enable the patient to sit comfortably before lying down. However, some tables may not lower, and a step stool may be necessary to use for the patient to climb up onto the table. The step stool should be sturdy and have a handle to grasp for support. If somebody accompanies the patient into the room, it is important to have a chair so he or she can sit comfortably during the exam to prevent syncope. The patient should be made as comfortable as possible during the exam, and after its completion the patient should be instructed to sit on the table before moving in case any dizziness is experienced.

Copyright © Mometrix Media. You have been licensed one copy of this document for personal use only. Any other reproduction or redistribution is strictly prohibited. All rights reserved.
This content is provided for test preparation purposes only and does not imply an endorsement by Mometrix of any particular political, scientific, or religious point of view.

Cardiac Arrest

Prior to the start of any exam, it is important to look at the patient's medical records to determine if he or she has an advance directive in place and if any do-not-resuscitate (DNR) orders exist. A patient can also have a DNR in place, even if an advance directive or living will have not been completed. If a patient has a DNR in place, then it has been decided by this individual to not undergo cardiopulmonary resuscitation if a cardiac event takes place. However, if working in a hospital setting and the patient does not have a DNR, the first thing the vascular technologist should do is facilitate a code. Many facilities have a code button in the room that the vascular technologist would push in order to activate the emergency response team. If the vascular lab is not in a hospital setting, then the first thing the technologist would do is dial 911 and call for the physician and crash cart. Regardless of the place of employment, medical personnel must be familiar with the policies and procedures in place when emergencies arise.

Copyright © Mometrix Media. You have been licensed one copy of this document for personal use only. Any other reproduction or redistribution is strictly prohibited. All rights reserved.
This content is provided for test preparation purposes only and does not imply an endorsement by Mometrix of any particular political, scientific, or religious point of view.

Physical Principles

Identifying Artifacts Related to Vascular Imaging

Calcifications

Response: Calcifications are the result of calcium buildup within the wall of the artery. During ultrasound exams, plaque that is calcified appears as bright echoes that will often display posterior shadowing. This acoustic shadowing can be problematic because it can hinder the examination of the entire artery. If the vascular technologist attempts to estimate the percentage of stenosis in the presence of shadowing, errors will likely occur during the calculations. However, it may be beneficial for the sonographer to try to change the method used to access the vessels that are difficult to visualize well when there is a significant amount of shadowing present. For example, the vascular technologist may be able to access the vessel from a more posterior or anterior approach.

Spectral Broadening

If a sonographer visualizes spectral broadening during a carotid duplex exam on a patient that does not have a stenosis or an occlusion, there are several things to consider. When using spectral Doppler, it is important to check that the sample volume is placed in the middle of the arterial lumen instead of being too close to either side of the blood vessel. Another factor that could contribute to spectral broadening without disease could be the size of the sample volume. The vascular technologist can control the sample size, and if it is too big the system could be picking up information within the middle of and near the wall of the artery. The Doppler angle should also be checked to make sure that the angle is 60 degrees or less.

Aliasing

Aliasing is considered an artifact that demonstrates an error in imaging. There are many steps that can be taken to eliminate signals that display aliasing. The first step that a vascular technologist should try is to adjust the PRF (velocity scale). When evaluating an artery, the blood flow is moving rapidly, so increasing the PRF may help unwrap the spectral display. This step increases the Nyquist limit, which is also known as the aliasing frequency, and is equal to half of the PRF. If this alone does not take care of aliasing, the baseline may be adjusted accordingly. Another helpful tip to eliminate aliasing is to switch to a lower frequency transducer or even find a window that isn't as deep. The angle of incidence could also be increased to help eliminate aliasing.

Aliasing and Flow Demonstrated below the Baseline

If a vascular technologist is using spectral analysis to determine the velocity of blood flow and notices flow velocities that are below the baseline, it can be assumed that this represents blood cells that are traveling in a direction away from the transducer. Aliasing is an error in imaging that can represent high-velocity flows that wrap around the baseline and appear as if they are moving in the opposite direction. An advantage of pulsed Doppler is that the user knows exactly where the

Copyright © Mometrix Media. You have been licensed one copy of this document for personal use only. Any other reproduction or redistribution is strictly prohibited. All rights reserved.
This content is provided for test preparation purposes only and does not imply an endorsement by Mometrix of any particular political, scientific, or religious point of view.

blood flow velocity is being sampled because one can adjust the gate. Color-flow Doppler allows information pertaining to the velocities to be superimposed on a gray-scale image. Color-flow Doppler is often used in conjunction with spectral waveforms to determine in which direction the blood is traveling.

Effect of Aliasing on Continuous-Wave Doppler

Aliasing is an error in imaging that occurs when using pulsed-wave Doppler if the waveform winds around the top or bottom of the display. Aliasing takes place when the Doppler shift is greater than the Nyquist limit, which is half of the PRF. Aliasing only occurs with pulsed Doppler (which includes color and pulsed-wave spectral Doppler). Using continuous-wave Doppler is one of many steps that a sonographer can use to overcome aliasing. Continuous-wave transducers contain two elements that constantly transmit and receive signals. There isn't any listening time with these transducers; therefore, there is no limit on the frequency shift. Continuous-wave Doppler is an essential tool to accurately measure high-velocity blood flow because aliasing never occurs with this modality.

Calculate, Perform, and Analyze Resistive Indices and Acceleration Times

Calculating the Resistive Index

Calculate the resistive index (RI) if the PSV of an arcuate renal artery is 41 cm/s and the EDV is 12 cm/s.

The resistive index (RI) is calculated during certain exams to measure how pulsatile blood flow is due to the peripheral resistance that is found in a more distal location than where the blood flow is being measured. The RI is calculated with the following formula: $\mathrm{RI} = \frac{\mathrm{PSV}-\mathrm{EDV}}{\mathrm{PSV}}$. By plugging the known values into the formula, we can calculate the RI as follows: $\frac{41-12}{41} = \frac{29}{41} = 0.71$.

If the RI is calculated during a renal arterial duplex, it is considered abnormal if the RI is greater than or equal to 0.7, and normal if the value is less than 0.7.

Helpfulness of Calculating the Acceleration Time

It can be helpful to calculate the acceleration time during an arterial study to discern if the patient's symptoms are due to inflow or outflow conditions. If an obstruction of the artery is present in the region of the blood vessel that is proximal to where the vascular technologist has the transducer, there will be a longer amount of time between the start of systole and the greatest peak velocity. On the other hand, the acceleration time will not be longer if the patient has a significant stenosis or occlusion in the region of the artery that is in a more distal location to where the artery is being interrogated. Notably, an example of inflow disease would be an aortoiliac stenosis because it refers to problems of blood traveling into the legs from the heart. An example of outflow disease would be a stenosis because blood is attempting to travel from the femoral artery to the rest of the lower extremity.

Copyright © Mometrix Media. You have been licensed one copy of this document for personal use only. Any other reproduction or redistribution is strictly prohibited. All rights reserved.
This content is provided for test preparation purposes only and does not imply an endorsement by Mometrix of any particular political, scientific, or religious point of view.

If the acceleration time of the CFA was calculated to be 145 msec, explain why this is considered to be an abnormal finding.

When evaluating the acceleration time of the CFA, it is considered to be abnormal if this number is greater than or equal to 133 msec. Because 145 msec is greater than 133 msec, the acceleration time of this particular patient is abnormal, and it correlates to significant disease of the iliac artery. To gain a better understanding of an abnormal finding, it is also important to study the appearance of the arterial waveform. The acceleration time is considered to be abnormal if there is a slow upslope from the beginning of systole to the maximum peak velocity. When there is a rapid upslope demonstrated from the beginning of systole to the maximum peak velocity, the acceleration time is considered to be normal.

Copyright © Mometrix Media. You have been licensed one copy of this document for personal use only. Any other reproduction or redistribution is strictly prohibited. All rights reserved.
This content is provided for test preparation purposes only and does not imply an endorsement by Mometrix of any particular political, scientific, or religious point of view.

Preparation, Documentation, and Communication

Adapt the Exam to the Clinical Setting and Patient Condition

Warm Room

The vascular technologist should make a considerable effort to keep the patient as comfortable as possible during any test that is performed, but this is especially important during an arterial exam to try to avoid or at least keep the effects of vasoconstriction of the arteries as minimal as possible. This includes making sure that the patient has changed into comfortable garments that fit them, if necessary, to having him or her positioned correctly on the exam table. Another important factor that may be overlooked during vascular exams is to set the temperature of the exam room to something that is pleasant enough so the patient isn't extremely cold, which is often the case in hospitals and outpatient facilities. If the patient complains of being cold, the heat should be turned up in the room and warm blankets can be offered.

Confirming the Medications

When patients are seen for exams, they are often asked to provide a list of medications that are currently being taken (to include prescription and over-the-counter medications). This list of medications is important in case of any type of reaction if more medications are to be administered. Serious reactions can occur when patients are already taking certain medications, so it is important to not mix them if they are contraindicated. Over-the-counter medications may also cause reactions, so it is important to list all of them (even herbal supplements and vitamins). Patients should also list any negative affects they have experienced from either prescription or over-the-counter medications because if they are allergic to medications it is important that they are not given those medications. Diphenhydramine (Benadryl) is a common medication that may need to be given in the radiology lab, but if the patient is allergic it must be avoided. It is also important to note if the patient is taking insulin or glucagon and if their kidneys are functioning normally because many exams require the use of contrast, which can be hard on the kidneys.

Review and Confirm Patient Information and Communicate the Exam Process

Correctly Identifying the Patient

Whether working in a hospital or outpatient clinic, it is the responsibility of the vascular technologist as well as the staff members that check patients in to make sure that the patient is correctly identified. It may be an easier task in a hospital setting because a patient is often given a wristband with their name, date of birth, and medical record number. This wristband should be checked by all personnel prior to the start of any exam. Some electronic medical records systems will require

Copyright © Mometrix Media. You have been licensed one copy of this document for personal use only. Any other reproduction or redistribution is strictly prohibited. All rights reserved.
This content is provided for test preparation purposes only and does not imply an endorsement by Mometrix of any particular political, scientific, or religious point of view.

the technologist to scan the wristband to confirm the identity of the patient. Not every outpatient clinic uses wristbands, but the vascular technologist should use at least two identifiers to determine that they have the correct patient. For example, the sonographer should ask the patient his or her full name along with their date of birth. If they have had prior imaging, it is important that the information matches previous exams or else the picture archive and communication system (PACS) will not be linked to the current exam. Furthermore, it is expensive to perform exams on the wrong patient, and it must be documented if the incorrect patient is scanned.

General Information on an Imaging Report

Just as ultrasound images must have important patient identifier information, the ultrasound report generated by the radiologist must also contain certain information. An ultrasound imaging report must have the patient's name, medical record number, date of birth, facility where the exam was performed, ordering physician, and the name of the physician reading the report. The final report should also list the procedure that was performed, the date of the exam, and the indications for completing it. The reading physician should also report if it is being compared with any prior studies, where they were performed, and the date. The radiologist should also include any proposed follow-up exams that are recommended and the time frame in which this imaging should take place.

When ultrasound guidance procedures are performed, the final report that is generated must have the following basic information: the patient's name and date of birth, medical record number, facility where the exam was performed, the time and date of the procedure, why it was ordered, and the ordering physician. Ultrasound guidance may be done by the radiologist, so the doctor that performed the procedure should be noted. It should also be documented in the report that the exam was explained to the patient and a consent form was signed. Important information that must be included are the specific location of the target, medications (as well as the amount used) that were used, the type and size of needle that was necessary, and the approach that the physician used. The reading physician should also comment on things such as the number of tissue specimens taken and how they were prepared to be sent off to pathology. If complications were present during the procedure, this should also be included. Pre- and postprocedure images should be taken and included in the report.

Document Preliminary Impression/Findings and Technical Limitations

Information Contained on Ultrasound Images

An ultrasound exam is considered as part of the patient's permanent medical records. Although every effort must be made to preserve the confidentiality of the patient, ultrasound images must have certain information, including the patient's name, date of birth, medical record number that is unique to that patient, the facility in which the exam was performed, and the date of the exam. Ultrasound images are also annotated and should include the anatomical structure being examined, the side of the patient being examined when applicable, as well as the imaging plane (sagittal, transverse, coronal). Measurements of normal and abnormal anatomy and

Copyright © Mometrix Media. You have been licensed one copy of this document for personal use only. Any other reproduction or redistribution is strictly prohibited. All rights reserved.
This content is provided for test preparation purposes only and does not imply an endorsement by Mometrix of any particular political, scientific, or religious point of view.

pathology should also be documented during the exam. If necessary, color and/or spectral Doppler should be performed and recorded. If the vascular technologist is saving information into a worksheet package on the machine, that information can also be printed out for the reading physician.

Preliminary Reports

Vascular technologists are often required to perform an exam such as a venous duplex exam or abdominal aortic ultrasound in which the ordering physician wants immediate results. Sometimes, positive exams such as a DVT or an aneurysm require prompt management for the patient. In cases of a critical finding, the reading physician will phone the ordering physician in addition to providing a written preliminary report that may be sent with the patient to the emergency department. It should be clearly marked that it is a preliminary report, and although it doesn't contain as much detail as the final report, it will contain information that is also found in the final report. These reports will still contain patient information and should also include who the radiologist spoke with and the time and date that the phone call was made to further document that the findings were communicated in a timely fashion.

Including Technically Limited Information

Often, vascular technologists are required to submit their own technologist impression worksheet or write-up for the reading physician. This worksheet is a great place to document any difficulties experienced during the ultrasound exam whether it is due to the patient's body habitus, the amount of bowel gas present, open sores or scabs that interfere with imaging, uncooperativeness of the patient, or if the patient refused the exam after it began. In some cases, existing pathology can also degrade the images that can be captured such as when shadowing is caused by calcifications during an arterial study. If the patient experienced an extreme amount of pain during an exam, which did not allow images to be completed per the normal protocol (such as compression images during a venous duplex exam), the technologist should also document this. It is sometimes helpful for the reading physician to scan or watch any concerning parts of the scan in real time to gain a better understanding of what is taking place. The radiologist should also document any limiting factors in the report.

Copyright © Mometrix Media. You have been licensed one copy of this document for personal use only. Any other reproduction or redistribution is strictly prohibited. All rights reserved.
This content is provided for test preparation purposes only and does not imply an endorsement by Mometrix of any particular political, scientific, or religious point of view.

Image Credits

Licensed Under CC BY 4.0 (creativecommons.org/licenses/by/4.0/)

Hepatofugal Flow: "Hepatofugal flow in portal vein" by Wikimedia user Mme Mim (https://commons.wikimedia.org/wiki/File:Hepatofugal_flow_in_portal_vein.jpg)

Licensed Under CC BY-SA 3.0 (creativecommons.org/licenses/by-sa/3.0/)

Aortic Dissection (Modified): "Aortic Dissection Echocardiogram" by Ksheka (https://commons.wikimedia.org/wiki/File:Aortic_dissection_-_Echocardiogram_-_Longitudinal_view.jpg)

Deep Vein Thrombosis: "DVTUS" by James Heilman, MD (https://commons.wikimedia.org/wiki/File:DVTUS.PNG)

Baker's Cyst (Modified): "Popliteal Cyst" by Nevit Dilmen (https://commons.wikimedia.org/wiki/File:Ultrasound_Scan_ND_0125091859_0930540.png)

Stenosis: "Internal carotid artery stenosis" by Wikimedia user Mme Mim (https://commons.wikimedia.org/wiki/File:Internal_carotid_artery_stenosis_in_ultrasound_near_occlusion.jpg)

Licensed Under CC BY-SA 2.5 (creativecommons.org/licenses/by-sa/2.5/)

Horseshoe Kidney: "Horseshoe Kidney Illustration" by Wikimedia user Prosyannikov (https://commons.wikimedia.org/wiki/File:Horseshoe_kidney_realistic.jpg)

Copyright © Mometrix Media. You have been licensed one copy of this document for personal use only. Any other reproduction or redistribution is strictly prohibited. All rights reserved.
This content is provided for test preparation purposes only and does not imply an endorsement by Mometrix of any particular political, scientific, or religious point of view.

How to Overcome Test Anxiety

Just the thought of taking a test is enough to make most people a little nervous. A test is an important event that can have a long-term impact on your future, so it's important to take it seriously and it's natural to feel anxious about performing well. But just because anxiety is normal, that doesn't mean that it's helpful in test taking, or that you should simply accept it as part of your life. Anxiety can have a variety of effects. These effects can be mild, like making you feel slightly nervous, or severe, like blocking your ability to focus or remember even a simple detail.

If you experience test anxiety—whether severe or mild—it's important to know how to beat it. To discover this, first you need to understand what causes test anxiety.

Causes of Test Anxiety

While we often think of anxiety as an uncontrollable emotional state, it can actually be caused by simple, practical things. One of the most common causes of test anxiety is that a person does not feel adequately prepared for their test. This feeling can be the result of many different issues such as poor study habits or lack of organization, but the most common culprit is time management. Starting to study too late, failing to organize your study time to cover all of the material, or being distracted while you study will mean that you're not well prepared for the test. This may lead to cramming the night before, which will cause you to be physically and mentally exhausted for the test. Poor time management also contributes to feelings of stress, fear, and hopelessness as you realize you are not well prepared but don't know what to do about it.

Other times, test anxiety is not related to your preparation for the test but comes from unresolved fear. This may be a past failure on a test, or poor performance on tests in general. It may come from comparing yourself to others who seem to be performing better or from the stress of living up to expectations. Anxiety may be driven by fears of the future—how failure on this test would affect your educational and career goals. These fears are often completely irrational, but they can still negatively impact your test performance.

Elements of Test Anxiety

As mentioned earlier, test anxiety is considered to be an emotional state, but it has physical and mental components as well. Sometimes you may not even realize that you are suffering from test anxiety until you notice the physical symptoms. These can include trembling hands, rapid heartbeat, sweating, nausea, and tense muscles. Extreme anxiety may lead to fainting or vomiting. Obviously, any of these symptoms can have a negative impact on testing. It is important to recognize them as soon as they begin to occur so that you can address the problem before it damages your performance.

Copyright © Mometrix Media. You have been licensed one copy of this document for personal use only. Any other reproduction or redistribution is strictly prohibited. All rights reserved.
This content is provided for test preparation purposes only and does not imply an endorsement by Mometrix of any particular political, scientific, or religious point of view.

The mental components of test anxiety include trouble focusing and inability to remember learned information. During a test, your mind is on high alert, which can help you recall information and stay focused for an extended period of time. However, anxiety interferes with your mind's natural processes, causing you to blank out, even on the questions you know well. The strain of testing during anxiety makes it difficult to stay focused, especially on a test that may take several hours. Extreme anxiety can take a huge mental toll, making it difficult not only to recall test information but even to understand the test questions or pull your thoughts together.

Effects of Test Anxiety

Test anxiety is like a disease—if left untreated, it will get progressively worse. Anxiety leads to poor performance, and this reinforces the feelings of fear and failure, which in turn lead to poor performances on subsequent tests. It can grow from a mild nervousness to a crippling condition. If allowed to progress, test anxiety can have a big impact on your schooling, and consequently on your future.

Test anxiety can spread to other parts of your life. Anxiety on tests can become anxiety in any stressful situation, and blanking on a test can turn into panicking in a job situation. But fortunately, you don't have to let anxiety rule your testing and determine your grades. There are a number of relatively simple steps you can take to move past anxiety and function normally on a test and in the rest of life.

Physical Steps for Beating Test Anxiety

While test anxiety is a serious problem, the good news is that it can be overcome. It doesn't have to control your ability to think and remember information. While it may take time, you can begin taking steps today to beat anxiety.

Just as your first hint that you may be struggling with anxiety comes from the physical symptoms, the first step to treating it is also physical. Rest is crucial for having a clear, strong mind. If you are tired, it is much easier to give in to anxiety. But if you establish good sleep habits, your body and mind will be ready to perform optimally, without the strain of exhaustion. Additionally, sleeping well helps you to retain information better, so you're more likely to recall the answers when you see the test questions.

Getting good sleep means more than going to bed on time. It's important to allow your brain time to relax. Take study breaks from time to time so it doesn't get overworked, and don't study right before bed. Take time to rest your mind before trying to rest your body, or you may find it difficult to fall asleep.

Along with sleep, other aspects of physical health are important in preparing for a test. Good nutrition is vital for good brain function. Sugary foods and drinks may give a burst of energy but this burst is followed by a crash, both physically and emotionally. Instead, fuel your body with protein and vitamin-rich foods.

Copyright © Mometrix Media. You have been licensed one copy of this document for personal use only. Any other reproduction or redistribution is strictly prohibited. All rights reserved.
This content is provided for test preparation purposes only and does not imply an endorsement by Mometrix of any particular political, scientific, or religious point of view.

Also, drink plenty of water. Dehydration can lead to headaches and exhaustion, especially if your brain is already under stress from the rigors of the test. Particularly if your test is a long one, drink water during the breaks. And if possible, take an energy-boosting snack to eat between sections.

Along with sleep and diet, a third important part of physical health is exercise. Maintaining a steady workout schedule is helpful, but even taking 5-minute study breaks to walk can help get your blood pumping faster and clear your head. Exercise also releases endorphins, which contribute to a positive feeling and can help combat test anxiety.

When you nurture your physical health, you are also contributing to your mental health. If your body is healthy, your mind is much more likely to be healthy as well. So take time to rest, nourish your body with healthy food and water, and get moving as much as possible. Taking these physical steps will make you stronger and more able to take the mental steps necessary to overcome test anxiety.

Mental Steps for Beating Test Anxiety

Working on the mental side of test anxiety can be more challenging, but as with the physical side, there are clear steps you can take to overcome it. As mentioned earlier, test anxiety often stems from lack of preparation, so the obvious solution is to prepare for the test. Effective studying may be the most important weapon you have for beating test anxiety, but you can and should employ several other mental tools to combat fear.

First, boost your confidence by reminding yourself of past success—tests or projects that you aced. If you're putting as much effort into preparing for this test as you did for those, there's no reason you should expect to fail here. Work hard to prepare; then trust your preparation.

Second, surround yourself with encouraging people. It can be helpful to find a study group, but be sure that the people you're around will encourage a positive attitude. If you spend time with others who are anxious or cynical, this will only contribute to your own anxiety. Look for others who are motivated to study hard from a desire to succeed, not from a fear of failure.

Third, reward yourself. A test is physically and mentally tiring, even without anxiety, and it can be helpful to have something to look forward to. Plan an activity following the test, regardless of the outcome, such as going to a movie or getting ice cream.

When you are taking the test, if you find yourself beginning to feel anxious, remind yourself that you know the material. Visualize successfully completing the test. Then take a few deep, relaxing breaths and return to it. Work through the questions carefully but with confidence, knowing that you are capable of succeeding.

Developing a healthy mental approach to test taking will also aid in other areas of life. Test anxiety affects more than just the actual test—it can be damaging to your

Copyright © Mometrix Media. You have been licensed one copy of this document for personal use only. Any other reproduction or redistribution is strictly prohibited. All rights reserved.
This content is provided for test preparation purposes only and does not imply an endorsement by Mometrix of any particular political, scientific, or religious point of view.

mental health and even contribute to depression. It's important to beat test anxiety before it becomes a problem for more than testing.

Study Strategy

Being prepared for the test is necessary to combat anxiety, but what does being prepared look like? You may study for hours on end and still not feel prepared. What you need is a strategy for test prep. The next few pages outline our recommended steps to help you plan out and conquer the challenge of preparation.

Step 1: Scope Out the Test

Learn everything you can about the format (multiple choice, essay, etc.) and what will be on the test. Gather any study materials, course outlines, or sample exams that may be available. Not only will this help you to prepare, but knowing what to expect can help to alleviate test anxiety.

Step 2: Map Out the Material

Look through the textbook or study guide and make note of how many chapters or sections it has. Then divide these over the time you have. For example, if a book has 15 chapters and you have five days to study, you need to cover three chapters each day. Even better, if you have the time, leave an extra day at the end for overall review after you have gone through the material in depth.

If time is limited, you may need to prioritize the material. Look through it and make note of which sections you think you already have a good grasp on, and which need review. While you are studying, skim quickly through the familiar sections and take more time on the challenging parts. Write out your plan so you don't get lost as you go. Having a written plan also helps you feel more in control of the study, so anxiety is less likely to arise from feeling overwhelmed at the amount to cover.

Step 3: Gather Your Tools

Decide what study method works best for you. Do you prefer to highlight in the book as you study and then go back over the highlighted portions? Or do you type out notes of the important information? Or is it helpful to make flashcards that you can carry with you? Assemble the pens, index cards, highlighters, post-it notes, and any other materials you may need so you won't be distracted by getting up to find things while you study.

If you're having a hard time retaining the information or organizing your notes, experiment with different methods. For example, try color-coding by subject with colored pens, highlighters, or post-it notes. If you learn better by hearing, try recording yourself reading your notes so you can listen while in the car, working out, or simply sitting at your desk. Ask a friend to quiz you from your flashcards, or try teaching someone the material to solidify it in your mind.

Copyright © Mometrix Media. You have been licensed one copy of this document for personal use only. Any other reproduction or redistribution is strictly prohibited. All rights reserved.
This content is provided for test preparation purposes only and does not imply an endorsement by Mometrix of any particular political, scientific, or religious point of view.

Step 4: Create Your Environment

It's important to avoid distractions while you study. This includes both the obvious distractions like visitors and the subtle distractions like an uncomfortable chair (or a too-comfortable couch that makes you want to fall asleep). Set up the best study environment possible: good lighting and a comfortable work area. If background music helps you focus, you may want to turn it on, but otherwise keep the room quiet. If you are using a computer to take notes, be sure you don't have any other windows open, especially applications like social media, games, or anything else that could distract you. Silence your phone and turn off notifications. Be sure to keep water close by so you stay hydrated while you study (but avoid unhealthy drinks and snacks).

Also, take into account the best time of day to study. Are you freshest first thing in the morning? Try to set aside some time then to work through the material. Is your mind clearer in the afternoon or evening? Schedule your study session then. Another method is to study at the same time of day that you will take the test, so that your brain gets used to working on the material at that time and will be ready to focus at test time.

Step 5: Study!

Once you have done all the study preparation, it's time to settle into the actual studying. Sit down, take a few moments to settle your mind so you can focus, and begin to follow your study plan. Don't give in to distractions or let yourself procrastinate. This is your time to prepare so you'll be ready to fearlessly approach the test. Make the most of the time and stay focused.

Of course, you don't want to burn out. If you study too long you may find that you're not retaining the information very well. Take regular study breaks. For example, taking five minutes out of every hour to walk briskly, breathing deeply and swinging your arms, can help your mind stay fresh.

As you get to the end of each chapter or section, it's a good idea to do a quick review. Remind yourself of what you learned and work on any difficult parts. When you feel that you've mastered the material, move on to the next part. At the end of your study session, briefly skim through your notes again.

But while review is helpful, cramming last minute is NOT. If at all possible, work ahead so that you won't need to fit all your study into the last day. Cramming overloads your brain with more information than it can process and retain, and your tired mind may struggle to recall even previously learned information when it is overwhelmed with last-minute study. Also, the urgent nature of cramming and the stress placed on your brain contribute to anxiety. You'll be more likely to go to the test feeling unprepared and having trouble thinking clearly.

So don't cram, and don't stay up late before the test, even just to review your notes at a leisurely pace. Your brain needs rest more than it needs to go over the information again. In fact, plan to finish your studies by noon or early afternoon the

Copyright © Mometrix Media. You have been licensed one copy of this document for personal use only. Any other reproduction or redistribution is strictly prohibited. All rights reserved.
This content is provided for test preparation purposes only and does not imply an endorsement by Mometrix of any particular political, scientific, or religious point of view.

day before the test. Give your brain the rest of the day to relax or focus on other things, and get a good night's sleep. Then you will be fresh for the test and better able to recall what you've studied.

Step 6: Take a Practice Test

Many courses offer sample tests, either online or in the study materials. This is an excellent resource to check whether you have mastered the material, as well as to prepare for the test format and environment.

Check the test format ahead of time: the number of questions, the type (multiple choice, free response, etc.), and the time limit. Then create a plan for working through them. For example, if you have 30 minutes to take a 60-question test, your limit is 30 seconds per question. Spend less time on the questions you know well so that you can take more time on the difficult ones.

If you have time to take several practice tests, take the first one open book, with no time limit. Work through the questions at your own pace and make sure you fully understand them. Gradually work up to taking a test under test conditions: sit at a desk with all study materials put away and set a timer. Pace yourself to make sure you finish the test with time to spare and go back to check your answers if you have time.

After each test, check your answers. On the questions you missed, be sure you understand why you missed them. Did you misread the question (tests can use tricky wording)? Did you forget the information? Or was it something you hadn't learned? Go back and study any shaky areas that the practice tests reveal.

Taking these tests not only helps with your grade, but also aids in combating test anxiety. If you're already used to the test conditions, you're less likely to worry about it, and working through tests until you're scoring well gives you a confidence boost. Go through the practice tests until you feel comfortable, and then you can go into the test knowing that you're ready for it.

Test Tips

On test day, you should be confident, knowing that you've prepared well and are ready to answer the questions. But aside from preparation, there are several test day strategies you can employ to maximize your performance.

First, as stated before, get a good night's sleep the night before the test (and for several nights before that, if possible). Go into the test with a fresh, alert mind rather than staying up late to study.

Try not to change too much about your normal routine on the day of the test. It's important to eat a nutritious breakfast, but if you normally don't eat breakfast at all, consider eating just a protein bar. If you're a coffee drinker, go ahead and have your normal coffee. Just make sure you time it so that the caffeine doesn't wear off right in the middle of your test. Avoid sugary beverages, and drink enough water to stay

Copyright © Mometrix Media. You have been licensed one copy of this document for personal use only. Any other reproduction or redistribution is strictly prohibited. All rights reserved.
This content is provided for test preparation purposes only and does not imply an endorsement by Mometrix of any particular political, scientific, or religious point of view.

hydrated but not so much that you need a restroom break 10 minutes into the test. If your test isn't first thing in the morning, consider going for a walk or doing a light workout before the test to get your blood flowing.

Allow yourself enough time to get ready, and leave for the test with plenty of time to spare so you won't have the anxiety of scrambling to arrive in time. Another reason to be early is to select a good seat. It's helpful to sit away from doors and windows, which can be distracting. Find a good seat, get out your supplies, and settle your mind before the test begins.

When the test begins, start by going over the instructions carefully, even if you already know what to expect. Make sure you avoid any careless mistakes by following the directions.

Then begin working through the questions, pacing yourself as you've practiced. If you're not sure on an answer, don't spend too much time on it, and don't let it shake your confidence. Either skip it and come back later, or eliminate as many wrong answers as possible and guess among the remaining ones. Don't dwell on these questions as you continue—put them out of your mind and focus on what lies ahead.

Be sure to read all of the answer choices, even if you're sure the first one is the right answer. Sometimes you'll find a better one if you keep reading. But don't second-guess yourself if you do immediately know the answer. Your gut instinct is usually right. Don't let test anxiety rob you of the information you know.

If you have time at the end of the test (and if the test format allows), go back and review your answers. Be cautious about changing any, since your first instinct tends to be correct, but make sure you didn't misread any of the questions or accidentally mark the wrong answer choice. Look over any you skipped and make an educated guess.

At the end, leave the test feeling confident. You've done your best, so don't waste time worrying about your performance or wishing you could change anything. Instead, celebrate the successful completion of this test. And finally, use this test to learn how to deal with anxiety even better next time.

Review Video: Test Anxiety
Visit mometrix.com/academy and enter code: 100340

Important Qualification

Not all anxiety is created equal. If your test anxiety is causing major issues in your life beyond the classroom or testing center, or if you are experiencing troubling physical symptoms related to your anxiety, it may be a sign of a serious physiological or psychological condition. If this sounds like your situation, we strongly encourage you to seek professional help.

Copyright © Mometrix Media. You have been licensed one copy of this document for personal use only. Any other reproduction or redistribution is strictly prohibited. All rights reserved.
This content is provided for test preparation purposes only and does not imply an endorsement by Mometrix of any particular political, scientific, or religious point of view.

Online Resources

Due to our efforts to try to keep this book to a manageable length, we've created a link that will give you access to all of your online resources:

mometrix.com/resources719/ardmsvt

It's Your Moment, Let's Celebrate It!

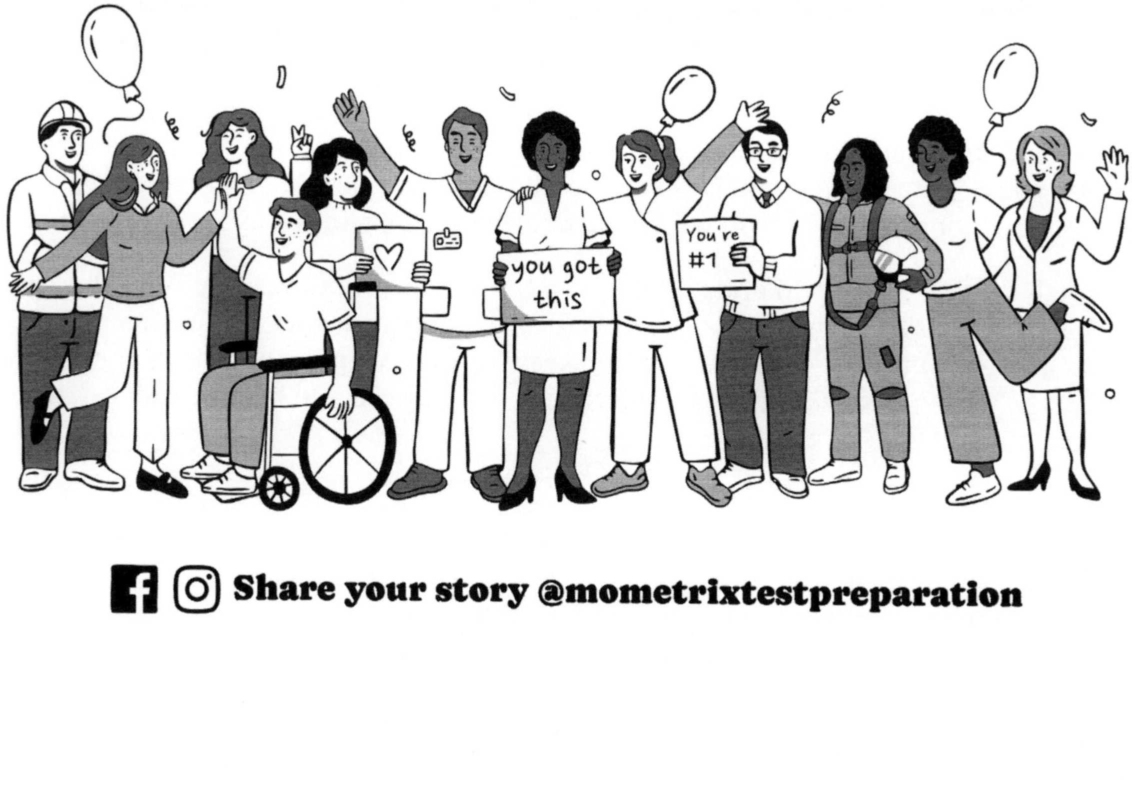

Share your story @mometrixtestpreparation

Copyright © Mometrix Media. You have been licensed one copy of this document for personal use only. Any other reproduction or redistribution is strictly prohibited. All rights reserved.
This content is provided for test preparation purposes only and does not imply an endorsement by Mometrix of any particular political, scientific, or religious point of view.